T0320565

COVID-19 and Emerging Environmental Trends

COVID-19 and Emerging Environmental Trends
A Way Forward

Joystu Dutta, Srijan Goswami, and
Abhijit Mitra

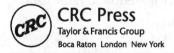

CRC Press
Taylor & Francis Group
Boca Raton London New York

CRC Press is an imprint of the
Taylor & Francis Group, an **informa** business

First edition published 2021
by CRC Press
6000 Broken Sound Parkway NW, Suite 300, Boca Raton, FL 33487-2742

and by CRC Press
2 Park Square, Milton Park, Abingdon, Oxon, OX14 4RN

Library of Congress Cataloging-in-Publication Data
Names: Dutta, Joystu, author. | Goswami, Srijan, author. | Mitra, Abhijit, author.
Title: COVID-19 and emerging environmental trends : a way forward / Joystu Dutta, Srijan Goswami, Abhijit Mitra.
Description: First edition. | Boca Raton, FL : CRC Press, 2021. | Includes index.
Identifiers: LCCN 2020038809 (print) | LCCN 2020038810 (ebook) |
ISBN 9780367623210 (hardback) | ISBN 9781003108887 (ebook)
Subjects: LCSH: COVID-19 (Disease) | COVID-19 (Disease)—Environmental aspects.
Classification: LCC RA644.C67 D88 2021 (print) | LCC RA644.C67 (ebook) |
DDC 614.5/92414—dc23
LC record available at https://lccn.loc.gov/2020038809
LC ebook record available at https://lccn.loc.gov/2020038810

ISBN: 978-0-367-62321-0 (hbk)
ISBN: 978-1-003-10888-7 (ebk)

Typeset in Times
by codeMantra

This book is dedicated to our parents

Contents

Preface

We know war destroys civilization and uproots the existence of mankind. A time was there when the whole planet was under the appalling shadow of atom bomb, but now it has become the ornaments of nation. Is it an adaptation? Well, we cannot come to the final conclusion. However, all that we can infer is that no dark phase lasts forever. The COVID-19 pandemic is undoubtedly an eclipse for all the nations of the world. With a death of around 573K people in a planet of 7 billion population, it is another war the nations are facing. It is no exaggeration to say that in this war, we still do not have any defense system that can destroy this micro species that took the lives of people worldwide. We are yet in an early stage regarding its origin, symptoms, and defense mechanisms. Surprisingly, the symptoms of the disease are exhibiting significant dynamicity. In this critical juncture, this book is an attempt to open the Pandora's box and reveals the virus in terms of its origin, nature, transmission, and effects. The lockdown phase, an attempt to break the transmission chain, however, showed some positive signs in terms of air and water quality, which have been depicted in this book with ground zero data. The book would not have arrived at the final stage without the constant support and assistance of our near and dear ones both in personal and in professional front. Our family stood as a pillar of support during these difficult times helping us to write the manuscript. We hope that the book written in a very lucid language would be able to draw attention of the readers of all ranks of the society.

Abhijit Mitra, Srijan Goswami, and Joystu Dutta

Authors

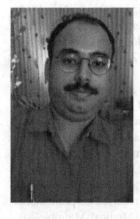

Joystu Dutta is an Assistant Professor in the Department of Environmental Science, Sant Gahira Guru University, Sarguja, a state university of the Government of Chhattisgarh. His main activities are teaching, research, and extension and engaged in supervising administrative activities in various capacities. He is a member of IUCN Commission of Ecosystem Management. He is a DST Inspire Fellow and also holds UNESCO scholarships besides UGC NET Lectureship in Environmental Sciences. He has written over 20 research papers in the national and international journals. He has participated in collaborative research projects with organizations such as JNU, Forest Research Institute Dehradun, Gujarat Institute of Desert Ecology, to name a few, as well as short-term consultancy-based projects with organizations such as Sahapedia and forest departments. Previously, he was with Reliance Foundation, CSR Wing of Reliance Industries Limited, Mumbai, as an Assistant Programme Manager (APM). He has more than 2 years of work experience in the field of rural development, advocacy, and corporate communications. He has also done internship as a Young Development Professional (YDP) with Reliance Foundation. He has received Gold Medals during his graduation and post-graduation studies and also received several accolades for the excellent professional achievements such as Vice Chancellor's Best Employee Award and Young Scientist Award by Indian Environmental Science Academy, among many others. He also voraciously writes in journals and newsletters and is in the Editorial Review Board of various national and international journals. Mr. Dutta loves to work with communities at grass root levels. During leisure, Joystu is busy reading story books, writing poems and plays, traveling to new places, and swimming. He is also an established stage actor and writes as well as direct plays for his students. His university team has received National Award from Digital India Program, Ministry of Information and Broadcasting, Government of India for the best play at the university level.

Currently, Mr. Dutta is pursuing his doctoral research in Environmental Toxicology besides engaging himself with Voice of Environment, a Guwahati-based NGO that works in the sector of environmental awareness and sustainable conservation approaches.

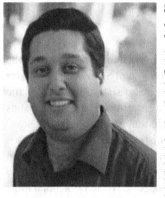

Srijan Goswami is the Founder Director of the Indian School of Complementary Therapy and Allied Sciences, Kolkata, India (Non-Government and Non-Profit Organization). Presently, he is the Guest Faculty of Immunology and Physiology at the Department of Zoology (PG courses), Serampore College, India. He worked as Assistant professor at the Department of Biotechnology and Molecular Biology, Institute of Genetic Engineering, Badu, India, till July 2018 and as a Lecturer at the Department of Computer Science, Webel Informatics Limited, Basirhat College Unit, India, till June 2016. Dr. Goswami is a Physician of Biochemic System of Medicine and also holds specialization in Medical Biotechnology and Clinical Nutrition. He received his professional training on Community Nutrition and Child Care, Medical Microbiology, and Medical Biochemistry from reputed medical colleges in Kolkata, India and holds a PGDSE from Webel, India. He has around 7 years of experience in the field of teaching and research and has written 20 research papers in the national and international journals. He has independently and successfully guided around ten undergraduate and postgraduate students to complete their research work and publications in the past 3 years. He acted as an Examination Superintendent for National Digital Literacy Mission at Pravda Infotech Pvt. Ltd (Basirhat), India, in 2016. He has qualified in PhD Entrance Examination conducted by the Department of Biotechnology, MAKAUT, in 2018. Dr. Goswami has received three Letters of Commendation for Global Community Services and Certificate of Honor for his contribution in the field of Science and Knowledge from the *International Journal of Agricultural Research, Sustainability and Food Sufficiency* (IJARSFS), *International Journal of Advances in Medical Sciences and Biotechnology* (IJAMSB), and *International Journal of Health, Safety and Environment* (IJHSE) in 2019 and 2020. The *Current Research in Nutrition and Food Science* (Enviro Research Group) and *Academia Scholarly Journals* have awarded him the Certificate of Excellence as a Reviewer in 2020. He is actively associated as Editorial Review Board Member of 15 international journals and holds the post of Honorary Vice-Principal and Head of the Department of Physiology at Shree Krishna Biochemic College, Kolkata, India. Currently, Dr. Goswami is pursuing his second professional MSc in Clinical Dietetics. His domain of expertise includes Molecular Biology, Medical Informatics, Clinical Nutrition, Immunonutrition, Mechanism of Drug Action, Nutraceuticals and Functional Foods, Holistic Science, and One Health.

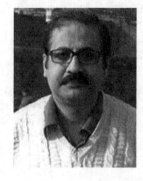

Abhijit Mitra is an Associate Professor and Former Head in the Department of Marine Science, University of Calcutta, India and has been active in the sphere of Oceanography since 1985. He obtained his PhD as a NET-qualified scholar in 1994 after securing Gold Medal in MSc (Marine Science) from the University of Calcutta. Since then, he joined Calcutta Port Trust and World Wildlife Fund (WWF) in various capacities to carry out research programs on environmental science, biodiversity conservation, and climate change, and carbon sequestration. Presently, Dr. Mitra is serving Techno India University as a Director of Research. He has to his credit about 553 scientific publications in various national and international journals and 42 books of postgraduate standards. He is presently the member of several committees like PACON International, IUCN, SIOS, etc. and has successfully completed about 19 projects on biodiversity loss in fishery sector, coastal pollution, alternative livelihood, climate change, and carbon sequestration. Dr. Mitra also visited as a faculty member and was invited as a speaker in several foreign universities of Singapore, Kenya, Oman, and USA. In 2008, Dr. Mitra was invited as a visiting fellow at the University of Massachusetts at Dartmouth, USA, to deliver a series of lecture on climate change. Dr. Mitra also successfully guided 38 PhD students. Presently, his domain of expertise includes Environmental Science, Mangrove Ecology, Sustainable Aquaculture, Alternative Livelihood, climate Change, and Carbon Sequestration.

Introduction to Coronaviruses and COVID-19

1

1.1 INTRODUCTION

In December 2019, a cluster of pneumonia incident was reported in the city of Wuhan, China. Some of the early cases of the transmission were reported to have started from a seafood and live animal market in Wuhan (WHO, 2020c). Investigations revealed that the disease is caused by a newly discovered member of the coronavirus family (Huang et al., 2019). The disease was named as COVID-19 (WHO, 2020b). The disease first spread within China and then to the rest of the world, which includes 216 countries, their areas, or territories. The World Health Organization (WHO) declared the outbreak a Public Health Emergency of International Concern on January 30, 2020. Table 1.1 represents the Coronavirus disease (COVID-19) outbreak situation of the top ten countries as of June 30, 2020.

TABLE 1.1   Coronavirus disease (COVID-19) outbreak situation of top ten countries as of June 30, 2020

REGION OF WORLD	CONFIRMED CASES	RECOVERED	DEATHS
Worldwide	1,0434,835	5,322,785	509,779
United States	2,679,961	825,781	128,692
Brazil	1,408,485	790,040	59,656
Russia	647,849	412,650	9320
India	566,840	334,821	16,893
United Kingdom	312,654	No Data	43,730
Peru	285,213	174,535	9677
Chile	279,393	241,229	5688
Spain	249,271	150,376	28,355
Italy	240,578	190,248	34,767
Iran	227,662	188,758	10,817

Source: news.google.com/covid 19, 2020.

1.2 CORONAVIRUS: DEFINITION, HISTORY, AND CLASSIFICATION

Coronaviruses are a family of viruses having RNA as their genetic material and possess the ability to cause diseases in mammals and birds. The members of the coronavirus family have the largest RNA genome (Dimmock et al., 2007). These viruses are known to cause infections of the respiratory tract in humans that range from mild (example: common cold) to life-threatening conditions (example: SARS, COVID-19, etc.). The name "Coronavirus" was assigned because of their morphological appearance as observed under the electron microscope (Almeida et al., 1967; Almeida et al., 1968; Almeida, 2008). The word "Corona" in coronavirus means "Crown" in Latin. Scientists named June Almeida and David Tyrrell was the first to observe and study three previously uncharacterized human respiratory viruses (Almeida et al., 1967) and named those viruses as "Coronaviruses" based on their appearance (Tyrrell et al., 2002). In November 1968, Almeida and Tyrrell along with their co-researchers first published (in print form) the term "coronavirus" in *Nature* (Almeida et al., 1968). Table 1.2 points out the major historical events related to the discovery of and subsequent research on coronaviruses.

TABLE 1.2 Major historical timelines of coronavirus research

YEAR OF IDENTIFICATION	DISCOVERY	NAME OF THE ACTUAL RESEARCHER OR RELATED REFERENCES
1930	Acute respiratory infections of domesticated chickens by infectious bronchitis virus (IBV)	**Referenced in:** Estola (1970).
1931	New respiratory infections of chicken	First reported by Arthur Schalk and M.C. Hawn. **Referenced in:** Fabricant (1998).
1937	Isolation and cultivation of Infectious Bronchitis Virus (IBV)	First isolated and cultivated by Fred Beaudette and Charles Hudson. **Referenced in** Decaro (2011).
1940s	Isolation of two animal coronaviruses • Mouse hepatitis virus (MHV) • Transmissible gastroenteritis virus (TGEV)	**Referenced in** McIntosh (1974).

During the above-mentioned time period, the researchers were not aware that IBV, MHV, and TGEV are related.

1960s	Discovery of human coronaviruses	**Referenced in** Kahn (2005); Mahase (2020).
1960	Isolation of novel common cold virus B814 at Common Cold Unit of the British Medical Research Council	E.C. Kendall, Malcom Byone, and David Tyrrell **Referenced in** Kendall et al. (1962); Richmond (2005).
1965	Successful cultivation of B814	Malcom Byone, and David Tyrrell **Referenced in** Tyrrell and Byone, et al. (1965).
1966	Isolation of novel common cold virus 229E at University of Chicago	Dorothy Hamre and John Procknow **Referenced in** Knapp, (n.d.); Hamre and Procknow et al. (1966).

(Continued)

TABLE 1.2 (Continued)   Major historical timelines of coronavirus research

YEAR OF IDENTIFICATION	DISCOVERY	NAME OF THE ACTUAL RESEARCHER OR RELATED REFERENCES
1967	Imaging study of B814 and 229E under electron microscope by June Almeida (Scottish Virologist)	**Referenced in** Almeida (2008); Almeida et al. (1967).
	June Almeida and colleagues provided the relationship between B814-229E and IBV	**Referenced in** Almeida et al. (1967).
1967	Researchers at the National Institute of Health (NIH) isolated OC43 (OC – Organ Culture).	**Referenced in** McIntosh et al. (1967).
1968	Introduction of the term "Coronavirus" and nomenclature of the family.	**Referenced in** Almeida et al. (1968).
2003	Detection of SARS-CoV	**Referenced in** Su et al., (2016); Zhu et al. (2020).
2004	Detection of HCoV NL63	
2005	Detection of HCoV HKU1	
2012	Detection of MERS-CoV	
2019	Detection of SARS-CoV-2	

David Baltimore introduced the Baltimore classification system in which viruses are grouped into families based on the type of their genetic material. According to Baltimore classification, the members of the Coronavirus family are grouped as Class 4. Viruses belonging to Class 4 possesses +ve sense single-stranded RNA (ssRNA). The +ve ssRNA is converted to its antisense RNA, which is then reconverted to +ve ssRNA (Dimmock et al., 2007). The Baltimore classification system is schematically represented in Figure 1.1.

The International Committee on Taxonomy of Viruses (ICTV), established in the late 1960s, has developed a taxonomic classification system for viruses. This uses the familiar systematic taxonomy scheme of Order, Family, Subfamily, and Genus. It does not emphasize on Kingdoms, Phyla, or Class of viruses within this scheme (Dimmock et al., 2007). On the basis of this taxonomy, SARS-CoV-2 is classified under Order – *Nidovirales*, Family – *Coronaviridae*, and Genus – *Betacoronavirus* (Rehman et al., 2020).

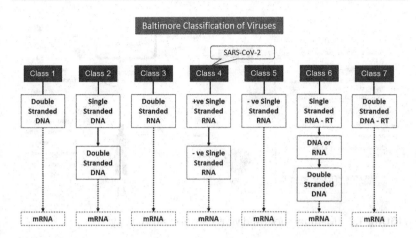

FIGURE 1.1   Baltimore classification of SARS-CoV-2.

1.3 BEHAVIOR OF VIRUSES

Before moving on to the details of COVID-19, it is important to understand the behavior of viruses. Viruses are neither living nor dead, so it is not possible to kill them. Viruses, when present in nature, stay as nonliving particles, but when the same virus gets access to host cells, it starts functioning as a living system. We may understand this behavior with an analogy of computers and memory sticks or flash drives. Memory sticks (pen drives) are portable plugging devices that can be attached to the USB port of a computer. They contain memory but do not have an operating system of their own, which means even if they have certain information stored in them, they cannot function autonomously. But when the same memory stick is connected to a computer (running on a proper operating system) through the USB port (the receptor), the program from the memory stick can be transferred to the computer. The operating system of the computer makes the information stored in the memory stick functional within the system. Viruses are equivalent to the memory sticks: they are not alive and do not have functional metabolism when present outside host cells. They are capsules containing the information to override and control the genetics and metabolism of host cells. So they can be thought of as invisible memory sticks floating all over the place and one of these memory sticks plugs itself into a host cell having appropriate receptors. The information present inside the virus then gets into the host cell just like on a computer. The information carried by the viruses then takes over the

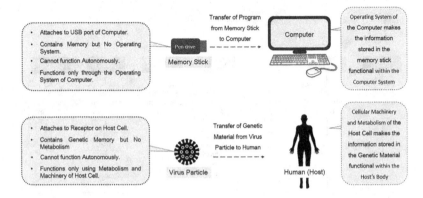

FIGURE 1.2 Memory sticks and virus particles: An analogy.

metabolic functions of the host cell and reprograms it to produce more virus particles. Accumulation of newly synthesized viral particles inside the host cells after being replicated results in the scattering of the virus particles into the system, which ultimately leads to cell death. These newly synthesized virus particles then infect other host cells and continue their lifecycle. And this process goes on like the domino effect (Lipton, 2020). Figure 1.2 shows the schematic representation of this concept.

1.4 ORIGIN OF THE NOVEL CORONAVIRUS nCoV-19

SARS-CoV-2 is a member of the family of coronaviruses specifically similar to the SARS virus. The SARS virus, also a coronavirus, appeared in 2002 and is known to cause severe acute respiratory syndrome. Researchers reported that the SARS virus used bats as their host; from the bats, the virus mutated in such a way that it gained the ability to infect another host (intermediate host). In general, coronaviruses are benign and do not significantly affect humans. But if this virus mutates enough inside primary and intermediate hosts (animal reservoir), they might gain the ability to cause severe diseases in humans. Severe acute respiratory syndrome is an example of this kind of incident. In 2012, another member of the coronavirus family, named as MERS virus, caused Middle East respiratory syndrome in humans. This time the MERS virus mutated from bats and jumped to camels (intermediate host). The virus acquired further mutations inside camels and got transmitted to humans. In 2019, SARS-CoV-2, a member of the coronavirus family, gained

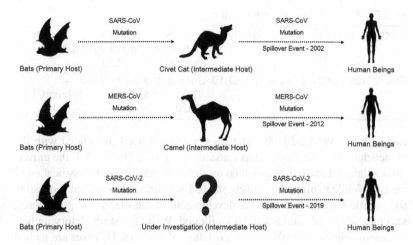

FIGURE 1.3 Three major spillover events.

mutation inside bats (primary host) and then jumped to an intermediate host (actual source of the intermediate host is still under investigation); it further mutated and gained the ability to infect human beings, causing COVID-19 (WHO, 2020e).

Analysis of the data revealed that coronaviruses acquired periodic mutations, which gave them the natural ability to overcome the species barrier. This ability of the coronaviruses allows them to be able to infect and survive inside a completely new species (host). This phenomenon is termed a *zoonotic spillover event* (see Figure 1.3). This term is used to indicate the situation when a virus has overcome the naturally occurring barriers necessary to "spill over" from one species to another. Though it is not easy to accurately predict the timeframe of a viral spill, researchers around the world are trying to identify a number of factors that may help in prediction of the events.

1.5 NOMENCLATURE OF NOVEL CORONAVIRUS nCoV-19 AND THE DISEASE

As reported by WHO, a new strain of coronavirus—thus called Novel Coronavirus (December 2019), or nCoV-19—was found to cause a cluster of pneumonia cases. Few months after this incident, official names were assigned to the 2019 Novel Coronavirus (nCoV-19) as well as the disease

TABLE 1.3   Highlights of Nomenclature Events

Official Name of the Virus: SARS-CoV-2	Given by the International Committee for the Taxonomy of Viruses (ICTV) on February 11, 2020
Official Name of the Disease: COVID-19	Given by the World Health Organization (WHO) on February 11, 2020.

caused by it (WHO, 2020b). There are various aspects associated with the nomenclature of a disease and its causative organism. The ICTV is the universal regulatory authority responsible for the nomenclature and classification of viruses. While naming the viruses, the ICTV mainly takes into consideration the genetic structure so that the development of the diagnostic procedures, vaccines, and medications can be facilitated. WHO is the regulatory authority responsible for the official nomenclature of diseases. Diseases are named to enable scientific research, design standard protocols for the understanding of transmissibility and severity, and strategize preventive measures, treatment, and management. On February 11, 2020, ICTV declared "Severe Acute Respiratory Syndrome Coronavirus 2 (SARS-CoV-2)" as the official name for the Novel Coronavirus (nCoV-19). So all the research papers and communications related to SARS-CoV-2 prior to February 11, 2020, refer to the name nCoV-19 and WHO declared that "Material published before the virus was officially named will not be updated unless necessary in order to avoid confusion" (WHO, 2020b). Based on the guidelines of World Organization for Animal Health, formerly Office International des Epizooties (OIE), and Food and Agriculture Organization of United States (FAO), WHO officially named the disease caused by SARS-CoV-2 as COVID-19 (Coronavirus Disease of 2019) on February 11th, 2020. There may be instances where WHO referred (or interchanged) SARS-CoV-2 as "the virus responsible for COVID-19" or "the COVID-19 virus" while communicating with the common public, which may lead to confusion regarding naming conventions. In this regard, WHO announced that the terminologies "virus responsible for COVID-19" and "the COVID-19 virus" are not intended as a replacement to the official name of the virus as declared by ICTV on February 11, 2020 (WHO, 2020b) (Table 1.3).

1.6 SYMPTOMS OF COVID-19

The incubation period can be considered as the time period between the infection of an individual by a pathogen and the manifestation of the illness or disease it causes. The average incubation period is 5–6 days but may also

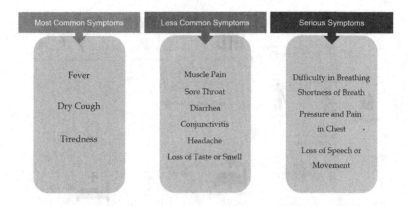

FIGURE 1.4 Symptoms associated with COVID-19. (www.who.int and www.cdc.gov, 2020.)

extend up to 14 days. The symptoms may vary from being asymptomatic to having a severe respiratory distress syndrome. The intensity of manifestation of symptoms is dependent on multiple factors (WHO, 2020d; CDC, 2020). The symptoms associated with COVID-19 are presented in Figure 1.4.

1.7 TRANSMISSION OF COVID-19

There are two basic ways by which an individual can get infected by SARS-CoV-2: one is through the "respiratory droplets," and the other is through "droplet nuclei" (WHO, 2020a). Respiratory droplets are droplet particles that are >5–10 μm in diameter, whereas droplet particles of size <5μm in diameter are called droplet nuclei (WHO, 2014). Several researchers have reported that respiratory droplets and contact routes are the primary modes of transmission between individuals (Liu et al., 2020; Chan et al., 2020; Li et al., 2020; Burke et al., 2020; WHO, 2020a). Transmission through droplets is possible when an individual is in close contact (generally within 1 m) with the infected person (See Figure 1.6). The infected person may transmit the virus through a cough or sneeze or sometimes just by talking (without protective masks), and as a result, the mucosa (nose and mouth) and conjunctiva (eyes) of the healthy person may get exposed to potentially infective respiratory droplets (Ong et al., 2020). The virus can also get transmitted through fomites (Ong et al., 2020). Fomites are the objects contaminated with infectious agents (in this case the SARS-CoV-2) and serve in their transmission. Therefore, direct contact with an infected individual and indirect contact with fomites are

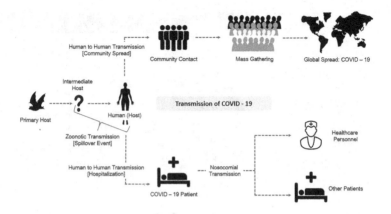

FIGURE 1.5 Sequence of transmission of COVID-19.

the major ways by which SARS-CoV-2 can get transmitted (See Figures 1.5 and 1.6). Sometimes, the droplet nuclei (containing the pathogen) remains in the air for a long period of time and gets transmitted to individuals over distances greater than 1 meter. This phenomenon is called *airborne transmission*. Airborne transmission of COVID-19 is possible under specific circumstances in which aerosol production is facilitated. Endotracheal intubation, noninvasive positive pressure ventilation, and disconnecting a patient from the ventilators are some of the situations (among many) that can lead

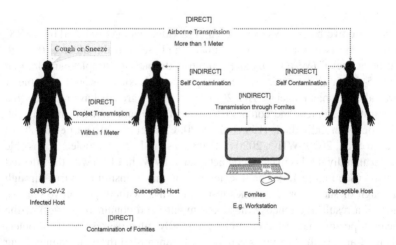

FIGURE 1.6 Transmission of COVID-19 through respiratory droplets, aerosols, and fomites.

to airborne transmission (WHO, 2020a). A group of researchers from China reported that COVID-19 may give rise to intestinal symptoms and that the viral particles may be present in the feces of the patient (Zhang et al., 2020). According to WHO, no report of fecal–oral transmission of COVID-19 has been reported until June 30, 2020 (WHO, 2020). Figure 1.5 represents the sequence of transmission of COVID-19.

REFERENCES

Almeida, J. (2008, June 26). "June Almeida (née Hart)." *British Medical Journal*, 336 (7659): 1511.1–1511. DOI:10.1136/bmj.a434. ISSN 0959-8138. PMC 2440895.

Almeida, J.D., Berry, D.M., Cunningham, C.H., Hamre, D., Hofstad, M.S., Mallucci, L., McIntosh, K., and Tyrrell, D.A. (1968, November). "Virology: Coronaviruses." *Nature*, 220 (5168): 650. Bibcode:1968Natur.220.650. doi:10.1038/220650b0. [T]here is also a characteristic "fringe" of projections 200 A long, which are rounded or petal shaped... This appearance, recalling the solar corona, is shared by mouse hepatitis virus and several viruses recently recovered from man, namely strain B814, 229E and several others.

Almeida, J.D., and Tyrrell, D.A. (1967, April). "The morphology of three previously uncharacterized human respiratory viruses that grow in organ culture." *The Journal of General Virology*, 1 (2): 175–178. DOI:10.1099/0022-1317-1-2-175. PMID 4293939.

Burke, R.M., Midgley, C.M., Dratch, A., et al. (2020). "Active monitoring of persons exposed to patients with confirmed COVID-19 — United States, January–February 2020." *Morbidity and Mortality Weekly Report*. DOI: 10.15585/mmwr.mm6909e1external icon.

Chan, J., Yuan, S., Kok, K. et al. (2020). "A familial cluster of pneumonia associated with the 2019 novel coronavirus indicating person-to-person transmission: a study of a family cluster." *Lancet*. DOI: 10.1016/S0140-6736(20)30154-9.

Centers for Disease Control and Prevention. (2020). Coronavirus Disease 2019 (COVID-19) – Symptoms of Coronavirus. Retrieved June 22, 2020, from https://www.cdc.gov/coronavirus/2019-ncov/symptoms-testing/symptoms.html.

Decaro, N. (2011). "Gammacoronavirus." In Tidona, C., Darai, G. (eds.). *Gammacoronavirus‡: Coronaviridae. The Springer Index of Viruses*. Springer. pp. 403–413. DOI:10.1007/978-0-387-95919-1_58. ISBN 978-0-387-95919-1. PMC 7176155.

Dimmock, N.J., Easton, A.J., and Leppard, K.N. (2007). *Introduction to Modern Virology*, 6th ed. Blackwell Publishing Ltd.

Estola, T. (1970). "Coronaviruses, a new group of animal RNA viruses." *Avian Diseases*, 14 (2): 330–336. DOI:10.2307/1588476. ISSN 0005-2086. JSTOR 1588476

Fabricant, J. (1998). "The early history of infectious bronchitis." *Avian Diseases*, 42 (4): 648–650. DOI:10.2307/1592697. ISSN 0005-2086. JSTOR 1592697.

Hamre, D., and Procknow, J.J. (1966, January). "A new virus isolated from the human respiratory tract." *Proceedings of the Society for Experimental Biology and Medicine. Society for Experimental Biology and Medicine*, 121 (1): 190–193. DOI:10.3181/00379727-121-30734. PMID 4285768.

Huang, C., Wang, Y., Li, X., et al. (2020). "Clinical features of patients infected with 2019 novel coronavirus in Wuhan, China." *Lancet*, 395: 497–506.

Kahn, J.S., and McIntosh, K. (2005, November). "History and recent advances in coronavirus discovery." *The Pediatric Infectious Disease Journal*, 24 (11 Suppl): S223–S227, discussion S226. DOI:10.1097/01.inf.0000188166.17324.60. PMID 16378050.

Kendall, E.J., Bynoe, M.L., and Tyrrell, D.A. (1962, July). "Virus isolations from common colds occurring in a residential school." *British Medical Journal*, 2 (5297): 82–86. DOI:10.1136/bmj.2.5297.82. PMC 1925312. PMID 14455113.

Knapp, A. (n.d.) "The secret history of the first coronavirus." *Forbes*. Retrieved May 06, 2020.

Li, Q., Guan, X., Wu, P., et al. (2020) "Early transmission dynamics in Wuhan, China, of novel coronavirus-infected pneumonia." *The New England Journal of Medicine* DOI: 10.1056/NEJMoa2001316.

Lipton, B. H., PhD (2020, March 30). Bruce Lipton on COVID-19, Coronavirus Pandemic & Evolution [Video] https://www.youtube.com/watch?v=oyijHfL-W7w&t=2728s Accessed on June 27, 2020.

Liu, J., Liao, X., Qian, S. et al. (2020). "Community transmission of severe acute respiratory syndrome coronavirus 2, Shenzhen, China, 2020." *Emerging Infectious Diseases*. DOI: 10.3201/eid2606.200239.

Mahase, E. (2020, April). "The BMJ in 1965." *British Medical Journal*. 369: m1547. doi:10.1136/bmj.m1547. PMID 32299810.

Merriam-Webster. (n.d.). Incubation period. In *Merriam-Webster.com dictionary*. Retrieved June 24, 2020, from https://www.merriam-webster.com/dictionary/incubation%20period.

McIntosh, K. (1974). "Coronaviruses: a comparative review." In Arber, W., Haas, R., Henle, W., Hofschneider, P.H., Jerne, N.K., Koldovský, P., Koprowski, H., Maaløe, O., and Rott, R. (eds.). *Current Topics in Microbiology and Immunology / Ergebnisse der Mikrobiologie und Immunitätsforschung. Current Topics in Microbiology and Immunology / Ergebnisse der Mikrobiologie und Immunitätsforschung*. Berlin, Heidelberg: Springer, 87. DOI:10.1007/978-3-642-65775-7_3. ISBN 978-3-642-65775-7.

McIntosh, K., Becker, W.B., and Chanock, R.M. (1967, December). "Growth in suckling-mouse brain of "IBV-like" viruses from patients with upper respiratory tract disease." *Proceedings of the National Academy of Sciences of the United States of America*, 58 (6): 2268–2273. Bibcode:1967PNAS...58.2268M. DOI:10.1073/pnas.58.6.2268. PMC 223830. PMID 4298953.

Ong, S.W., Tan, Y.K., Chia, P.Y., et al. (2020, March 4) "Air, surface environmental, and personal protective equipment contamination by severe acute respiratory syndrome coronavirus 2 (SARS-CoV-2) from a symptomatic patient." *The Journal of the American Medical Association* [Epub ahead of print].

Rehman, S.U., Shafique, L., Ihsan, A., and Liu, Q. (2020). "Evolutionary trajectory for the emergence of novel coronavirus SARS-CoV-2." *Pathogens*, 9(3), 240. DOI:10.3390/pathogens9030240.

Richmond, C. (2005, June 18). "David Tyrrell." *British Medical Journal*, 330 (7505): 1451. DOI:10.1136/bmj.330.7505.1451. PMC 558394

Su, S., Wong, G., Shi, W., et al. (2016, June). "Epidemiology, genetic recombination, and pathogenesis of coronaviruses." *Trends in Microbiology*, 24 (6): 490–502. DOI:10.1016/j.tim.2016.03.003. PMC 7125511. PMID 27012512.

Tyrrell, D.A., Byone, M.L. (1965, June). "Cultivation of a novel type of common-cold virus in organ cultures." *British Medical Journal*, 1 (5448): 1467–1470. DOI:10.1136/bmj.1.5448.1467. PMC 2166670. PMID 14288084.

World Health Organization. (2014). *Infection Prevention and Control of Epidemic- and Pandemic-Prone Acute Respiratory Infections in Health Care*. Geneva: World Health Organization. https://apps.who.int/iris/bitstream/handle/10665/112656/9789241507134_eng.pdf?sequence=1.

World Health Organization. (2020a). Modes of Transmission of Virus Causing COVID-19 implications for IPC Precautions Recommendations. Retrieved June 22, 2020, from https://www.who.int/news-room/commentaries/detail/modes-of-transmission-of-virus-causing-covid-19-implications-for-ipc-precaution-recommendations.

World Health Organization. (2020b). Naming the Coronavirus Disease (COVID-19) and the Virus that Causes it. Retrieved June 24, 2020, from https://www.who.int/emergencies/diseases/novel-coronavirus-2019/technical-guidance/naming-the-coronavirus-disease-(covid-2019)-and-the-virus-thatcauses-it.

World Health Organization. (2020c). *Report of the WHO-China Joint Mission on Coronavirus Disease 2019 (COVID-19) 16–24 February 2020 [Internet]*. Geneva: World Health Organization. Available from https://www.who.int/docs/default-source/coronaviruse/who-china-joint-mission-on-covid-19-final-report.pdf.

World Health Organization. (2020d). Symptoms of COVID-19. Retrieved June 22, 2020, from https://www.who.int/emergencies/diseases/novel-coronavirus-2019/question-and-answers-hub/q-a-detail/q-a-coronaviruses#:~:text=symptoms.

Zhang, Y., Chen, C., Zhu, S. et al. (2020). "Isolation of 2019-nCoV from a stool specimen of a laboratory-confirmed case of the coronavirus disease 2019 (COVID-19)." *China CDC Weekly*, 2(8): 123–124. (In Chinese).

Zhu, N., Zhang, D., Wang, W., et al. (2020, February). "A novel coronavirus from patients with pneumonia in China, 2019." *The New England Journal of Medicine*, 382 (8): 727–733. doi:10.1056/NEJMoa2001017. PMC 7092803. PMID 31978945.

Biology of Coronaviruses with Special Reference to SARS-CoV-2

2

2.1 INTRODUCTION

The basic understanding of origin and development of coronavirus infection needs a clear study of pathogen biology. The fundamental structural and functional characteristics of the pathogen including life cycle and pathophysiology are discussed in this chapter. Research related to novel coronavirus strain SARS-CoV-2 or nCoV-2019 is emerging and rapidly evolving with new findings every day. This section discusses the established scientific communication until June 2020 after the discovery of the novel strain in January 2020. It is to be understood that similar findings might rapidly change in the upcoming days and open an altogether new vista in front of us with a deeper understanding and groundbreaking research on the virulent strain.

1. **Structure and Function of the Pathogen**
2. **The Lifecycle of the Pathogen** – Mechanism of entry, replication of genome, assembly of viral particles, and formation of viral progeny
3. **Pathophysiology** – The disordered physiological processes associated with disease or injury.

The above concepts would provide an understanding of how the organisms function and how the structures and functions are modified during the course of the disease. Understanding of lifecycle and underlying biochemical processes of the pathogen helps in designing the specific sophisticated diagnostic tests to facilitate the healthcare professionals to efficiently examine the patients. Most importantly, it helps in understanding the underlying biochemical pathways that can be used to develop targeted therapies.

2.2 SARS-CoV-2 STRUCTURE AND FUNCTION

2.2.1 Basic Structure of SARS-CoV-2

The SARS-CoV-2 has a spherical body along with various types of proteins on its outer surface. Some of these membrane proteins when studied closely under an electron microscope appear to be having a structure like "a crown." This crown-like appearance is the reason behind the name "coronavirus" because in *Latin*, the word "*corona*" means "a crown." This crown-like spike structures are common to all the representative members of coronavirus family. There are also various kinds of structural proteins that are present on the external surface of the coronaviruses (Astuti and Ysrafil, 2020). Spike protein (S), envelope protein (E), membrane protein (M), and nucleocapsid protein (N) are the four major structural proteins on the outer surface of SARS-CoV-2 that are similar to other coronaviruses (see Figure 2.2). Let us now understand each of these four proteins in detail.

2.2.1.1 Spike Protein

Spike protein or S-protein allows coronaviruses to attach to the host cell membrane. The fundamental structure of the S-protein is composed of two major subunits, namely subunit-1 (S1) and subunit-2 (S2). S1, also known as the receptor-binding domain (see Figure 2.1), helps the coronaviruses to bind to the host cell receptors (UniProtKB-P59594, 2020). In the case of SARS-CoV-2, the receptor-binding domain recognizes a specific receptor angiotensin-converting enzyme receptor-2 (ACE-2). Inside the human body, these ACE-2 receptors are located in the lungs, heart, kidneys, intestine, blood vessels, etc. The affinity of the receptor-binding domain of SARS-CoV-2 for ACE-2 has been found to be 20 times higher compared to

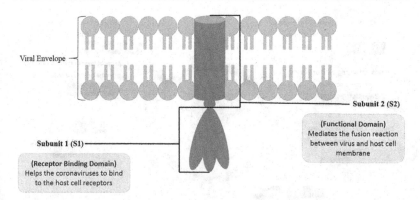

FIGURE 2.1 Basic structure of SARS-CoV-2 spike protein (S) (UniProtKB-P59594, 2020).

the normal SARS virus. This increased affinity makes the virus more infective. The second functional portion is known as S2 (see Figure 2.1), which mediates the fusion reaction between the virus and the host cell membrane (UniProtKB-P59594, 2020). The researchers reported that the S2 subunit undergoes several conformational changes to facilitate the successful membrane fusion (Chan et al., 2020). The sequential conformational changes promote the alignment and subsequent fusion of viral and host cell membranes (UniProtKB-P59594, 2020). Because of the critical roles they play in binding to target cells and mediating the entry, both S1 and S2 are regarded as the fundamental factors in relation to the designing of vaccines and also for creating synthetic drugs for the treatment of COVID-19.

2.2.1.2 Membrane Protein

Membrane proteins or M-proteins are the most abundant structural protein present on the surface of coronaviruses (see Figure 2.2), which determine the shape of the viral envelope (Chan et al., 2020). This protein is important because it acts as the central organizer for the assembly of coronaviruses, and it also interacts with other structural proteins during the process (UniProtKB-P59596, 2020).

2.2.1.3 Envelope Protein

Envelope protein or E-protein is the smallest among the four major structural proteins present on the surface of coronaviruses (see Figure 2.2), which performs several critical roles. First, it helps in the assembly and release of

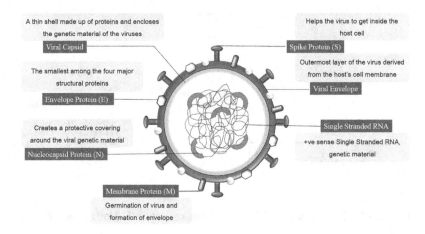

FIGURE 2.2   Basic structure of SARS-CoV-2.

viruses from host cells. Second, during viral replication, it is largely located at the regions of intracellular trafficking, for example, near endoplasmic reticulum and Golgi apparatus (Chan et al., 2020). So, both membrane and envelope proteins play an integral role in transforming the host cell apparatus into viral workshops where virus and host cells work together for making new viral particles (UniProtKB-P59637, 2020).

2.2.1.4 Viral Envelope

As shown in Figure 2.2, the viral envelope is present just under the surface proteins, which is the outermost layer of the virus derived from the host cell membrane. Since the host cell membrane is made up of phospholipids and proteins, the fundamental composition of the viral envelope is as same as the host cell membrane. The only difference is that in viruses, these membrane structures are incorporated with viral glycoproteins instead of host cell glycoproteins (Chan et al., 2020). The phospholipid–protein complex of the viral envelope gets denatured when treated with soap, which in turn destroys the virus. This is the reason that the World Health Organization recommended thorough handwashing with soap as an important preventive measure.

2.2.1.5 Viral Capsid

The capsid is located just below the viral envelope (see Figure 2.2). It is a thin shell made up of proteins and encloses the genetic material of the viruses (Chan et al., 2020).

2.2.1.6 Nucleocapsid Protein

The nucleocapsid proteins or N-proteins are present in association with the single-stranded RNA of the virus (see Figure 2.2). They are located below the capsid and create a protective covering around the viral genetic material. Nucleocapsid plays various critical roles in the virus life cycle (Chan et al., 2020). First, it provides protection to viral particles by inhibiting the host's defense mechanisms. Second, it assists viral RNA in replicating itself. Third, it aids in the generation of new viral particles (UniProtKB-59595, 2020).

2.2.2 Basic Structure of Genetic Material of SARS-CoV-2

The members of the coronavirus family possess a large genome containing approximately 30,000 nucleotides (29,891 nucleotides per initial investigation reports revealed by Chan et al., 2020). With a total G+C content of 38%, the genome is capable of synthesizing around 9860 amino acids (Chan et al., 2020). According to the Baltimore classification of viruses, coronaviruses belong to "Class-4," which means these viruses have positive-sense single-stranded RNA (+ve ssRNA) as their genetic material (Dimmock et al., 2007). The genetic material of coronaviruses is single stranded, linear chain, positive-sense structure having a 5′ cap and 3′ poly-A tail (see Figure 2.3). One important feature is that SARS-CoV-2 lacks the hemagglutinin–esterase (HE) gene in comparison with other coronaviruses (Chan et al., 2020). Considering from the 5′ end of the genetic material, there is an array of

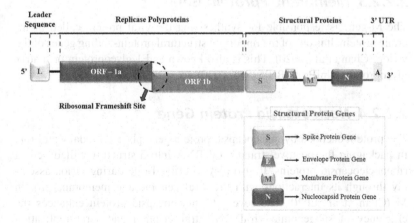

FIGURE 2.3 Basic structure of SARS-CoV-2 genome.

numerous structural components and functional genes; some of them are 5′-leader sequence, open reading frame 1a (ORF-1a), open reading frame 1b (ORF-1b), ribosomal frameshift site (present at the junction of ORF-1a and ORF-1b), S-gene, E-gene, M-gene, N-gene, and 3′ untranslated region (3′ UTR). ORF-1a and ORF-1b along with the ribosomal frameshift site fall under the group of genes that encode replicase polyproteins (also known as nonstructural proteins or nsps), and S, E, M, and N belong to the group of genes coding for the structural proteins (Swiss Institute of Bioinformatics, 2020). Figure 2.3 demonstrates the basic arrangement of major structural components and functional genes of SARS-CoV-2.

2.2.2.1 Spike Protein Gene

The S-gene is responsible for synthesizing the most important viral protein on SARS-CoV-2 called spike protein, the location and function of which are discussed in brief in Section 2.2.2.1 (UniProtKB-P59594, 2020). This par- ticular gene generates two distinct proteins named as spike proteins S1 and S2, which make up the intact spike protein characteristic of the coronaviruses (Chan et al., 2020).

2.2.2.2 Envelope Protein Gene

The E-gene is responsible for synthesizing an important viral protein called enve- lope protein (Chan et al., 2020). It interacts with M-protein and nucleoprotein in various processes during the lifecycle of SARS-CoV-2 (UniProtKB-P59637, 2020).

2.2.2.3 Membrane Pprotein Gene

The M-gene is responsible for synthesizing the viral protein called mem- brane protein. It is one of the important structural protein-coding genes of the virion (Chan et al., 2020). This is also known as E1 glycoprotein or matrix glycoprotein (UniProtKB-P59596, 2020).

2.2.2.4 Nucleocapsid Protein Gene

The protein encoded by nucleocapsid protein gene plays a fundamental role in packaging the positive-strand viral RNA into a structure called helical ribonucleocapsid proteins. It also plays a critical role during virion assem- bly through its interactions with the viral genome and membrane protein M (Chan et al., 2020). Moreover, the nucleocapsid protein enhances the efficiency of subgenomic viral RNA transcription and viral replication (UniProtKB-59595, 2020).

2.3 LIFECYCLE OF SARS-CoV-2

Like any other viruses, the members of the coronavirus family also require a host cell for their multiplication. Interaction with the host cell is necessary for gaining an entry so that the host's machinery can be utilized for the synthesis of viral particles. This section describes, in brief, the lifecycle of SARS-CoV-2. The lifecycle of coronaviruses is divided into three basic steps (Lim et al., 2016; Fehr et al., 2015):

1. Attachment and entry of a viral particle
2. Replication and transcription of the viral genetic material
3. Assembly and release of the viral particle

2.3.1 Attachment and Entry

It is known that SARS-CoV-2 spreads mainly by respiratory droplets through cough or sneeze, which aerosolizes the virus allowing it to enter into the nasal and oral cavity. SARS-CoV-2 can enter deep inside the lungs and damage the alveolar epithelial cells by replicating inside it, a property similar to other members of the family, such as SARS-CoV and MERS-CoV. The studies have shown that the multiplication of viral particles occurs within the epithelial cells of the upper respiratory tract (WHO, 2020). Angiotensin-converting enzyme-2 (ACE-2) and transmembrane serine protease 2 (TMPRSS 2), the two major enzymes present on the host cell membrane, are important for attachment and entry of viral particles (Lim et al., 2016; Fehr et al., 2015) (see Figure 2.4). The SARS-CoV-2 uses its spike proteins to bind to these ACE-2 receptors present on the host cell membrane. Once the S-protein recognizes the ACE-2 receptor, another important enzyme on the host cells called transmembrane serine protease 2 (TMPRSS 2) present near the ACE-2 receptors activates the S-protein. Following the activation by TMPRSS2, the S-protein binds to the ACE-2 receptor thus forming spike protein–ACE-2 receptor complex. The formation of spike protein–ACE-2 receptor complex promotes the fusion of viral envelope with the host cell membrane and results in subsequent endocytosis of the virus particle (Shang et al., 2020). Endocytosis is the process by which viruses enter the cells after being surrounded by an area of the host cell membrane, which then buds off inside the cell and forms a vesicle. The genomic RNA is then released into the host's cytoplasm (Lim et al., 2016; Fehr et al., 2015).

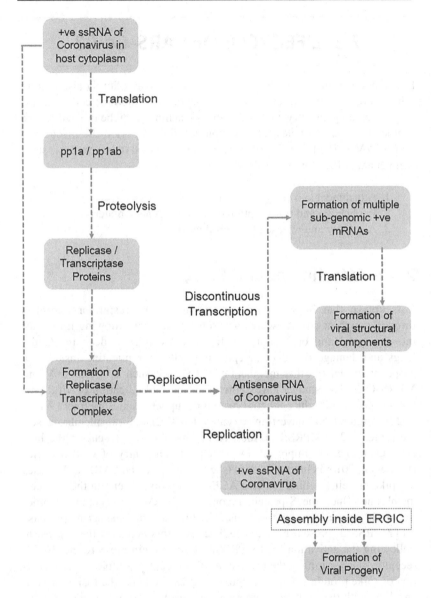

FIGURE 2.4 Schematic representation of SARS-CoV-2 replication cycle.

2.3.2 Replication and Transcription of Viral Genetic Material

The virus uses the host's ribosomes and enzymes for replicating the viral genomic RNA and also for translating viral genomic RNA into proteins. Consequently, virus-specific mRNA and proteins are synthesized inside the cytoplasm of host cells (Lim, 2016). The replication cycle of coronaviruses undergoes two important biochemical mechanisms.

- Ribosome frame shifting during genome translation: This can be observed during the initial production of polyproteins, which are actually used to generate most of the protein machinery of the replisome or transcriptosome.
- Synthesis of both genomic and multiple subgenomic RNA species.

The hallmark of the coronavirus transcription process is the production of many subgenomic mRNAs. Subgenomic mRNAs are different sized mRNAs that are created from the original RNA genome (Dimmock et al., 2007). Figure 2.5 indicates how all the biochemical reaction takes place inside the host cell after the release of viral genomic RNA. The viral genomic RNA utilizes the host cell machinery primarily the ribosomes for translating the viral genomic RNA strand in order to generate several structural and functional proteins essential for the virus lifecycle. Once the virus gets into the host cell, RNA-dependent RNA polymerase (RdRp) is produced by the transcription of original viral genomic RNA. The coronavirus utilizes RNA-dependent RNA synthesis to generate mRNAs to be transcribed by the host cell machinery. As the genomic RNA of the coronavirus undergoes translation utilizing the host ribosomes, two important polyproteins such as polyprotein-1a (pp1a) and polyprotein-1ab (pp1ab) (among many) are synthesized. These two major polyproteins are synthesized through frame shifting during translation and are further proteolyzed into numerous smaller proteins and play a critical role in viral replication and transcription (Fehr et al., 2015). So the proteins involved in replication are called replicase complex, whereas the proteins involved in transcription are called transcriptase complex. All these proteins combine with viral genomic RNA (sense strand) and facilitate replication. When the +ve ssRNA of the coronavirus replicates, an antisense RNA is produced. The conversion of the sense RNA into antisense RNA plays a significant role in the lifecycle of the virus. The antisense RNA is important because:

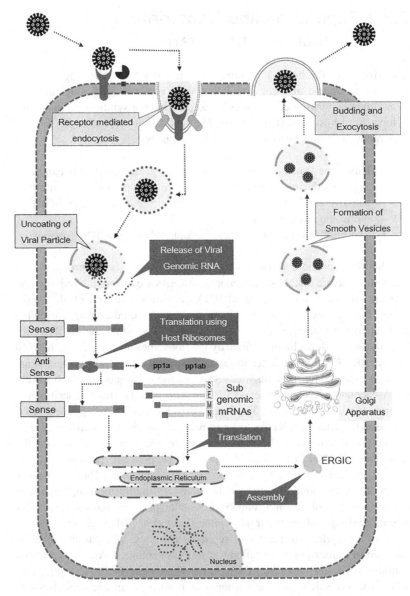

FIGURE 2.5   Schematic representation of SARS-CoV-2 lifecycle.

- It can be replicated back to sense RNA, which is essentially the same thing that came in with the parent virus during uncoating (Dimmock et al., 2007).

- This antisense RNA can be transcribed through a method called discontinuous transcription. Discontinuous transcription of anti-sense RNA generates a diverse range of mRNAs that can then be translated into different proteins (Dimmock et al., 2007).

2.3.3 Assembly and Release of Viral Particle

The assembly of newly synthesized viral particles begins with the systematic aggregation of +ve ssRNA and viral structural components (Lim, 2016). The assembly of newly synthesized coronavirus particles is accomplished through the budding of nucleocapsid through membranes early in the secretory pathway from the endoplasmic reticulum to the Golgi intermediate compartment or ERGIC. The contribution of the host cell during this process (in relation to SARS-CoV-2) is still under investigation. The M-protein also interacts with E-protein and S-protein to complete the assembly of the mature virus particles. Studies have shown that M-protein controls and regulates the viral assembly and mediates the budding of newly synthesized virus particles (Neuman et al., 2011). Following the assembly and budding, the newly assembled viral particles are transported in vesicles and eventually released by exocytosis.

2.4 PATHOPHYSIOLOGY

The viral particle inhaled through the nose or mouth enters the trachea or windpipe. Once SARS-CoV-2 gets into the respiratory system, it attacks the alveoli, which are responsible for the exchange of oxygen and carbon dioxide between the blood and atmosphere. Alveolus possesses two types of cells:

- **Type-I pneumocytes** – perform gas exchange.
- **Type-II pneumocytes** – involve in the production of surfactants. Surfactants decrease the surface tension within the alveoli and reduce the collapsing pressure.

SARS-CoV-2 enters the inner surface of alveoli and attacks the Type-II pneumocytes. After entering the host cell, the viral particle replicates and proliferates. These events result in the destruction of Type- II pneumocytes. The SARS-CoV-2 infection leads to a spectrum of severe complications such as pneumonia, acute respiratory distress syndrome (ARDS), consolidation, sepsis, septic shock, multisystem organ failure, and even death.

2.4.1 Pneumonia to Acute Respiratory Distress Syndrome: Underlying Cause

The damaged Type-II pneumocytes release specific inflammatory mediators, which are responsible for triggering and stimulating the macrophages. Stimulated macrophages secrete specific cytokines such as interleukin-1 (IL-1), interleukin-6 (IL-6), and tumor necrosis factor-α (TNF-α). These cytokines reach the bloodstream and cause the endothelial cells to undergo dilation. This cytokine action causes smooth muscle to dilate and increase the capillary permeability by contraction of endothelial cells. Consequently, the plasma starts flowing out and leaking into interstitial space and potentially into alveoli. Accumulation of fluid results in the compression of alveoli. Some of the fluid may try to enter into alveoli, and if a certain concentration of fluid enters alveoli, it leads to a condition called alveolar edema. Alveolar edema leads to the drowning out of the surfactants, which results in increased surface tension. As the surface tension increases, the collapsing pressure also increases, and as a result, the alveoli collapse, which is termed as alveolar collapse. The accumulation of a significant amount of fluid around the alveoli impairs the alveolar membrane (respiratory membrane), which results in decreased gas exchange. Decreased gas exchange leads to hypoxemia, which can be indicated as increased work of breathing (acute respiratory distress syndrome) (OpenWHO, 2020; Lim et al., 2016; Shang et al., 2020; Yuki et al., 2020; Mason, 2020; Fehr et al., 2015; Abbas et al., 2004).

2.4.2 Cough with Mucus in Patients with ARDS: Consolidation

All these inflammatory mediators also attract and bring in a number of neutrophils inside alveoli and try to destroy the virus. Destruction of the viruses by the inflammatory mediators results in the generation of reactive oxygen species (ROS) and proteases. ROS may destroy the viruses, but it also damages the Type-I and Type-II pneumocytes in the process. Damage caused to the Type-I and Type-II pneumocytes results in the lowering of gas exchange and increases the surface tension inside alveoli. Fluids, proteins, and cellular debris get accumulated at the center of the alveolus, which results in overcrowding inside the alveoli and in turn leads to consolidation. Consolidation refers to the pathological alteration of lung tissue from an aerated condition to one of a solid consistency (Merriam-Webster, 2020). This consolidation alters the rate of gas exchange leading to hypoxemia, which results in cough with mucus (OpenWHO, 2020; Lim et al., 2016; Shang et al., 2020; Yuki et al., 2020; Mason, 2020; Fehr et al., 2015; Abbas et al., 2004).

2.4.3 Reason behind High Body Temperature (Pyrexia), Increased Heart Rate (Tachycardia), and Increased Respiratory Rate (Tachypnea)

A significant amount of IL-1 and IL-6 can get transported from blood to the central nervous system. The hypothalamus, a very important part of the central nervous system, controls temperature. IL-1 and IL-6 signal the hypothalamus to release specific prostaglandins that increase the body temperature (fever/pyrexia). Again, a decrease in the partial pressure of oxygen inside the patient's body stimulates the chemoreceptors and triggers a reflex of the sympathetic nervous system (stimulated), which increases patient's respiratory rate (tachypnea) and heart rate (tachycardia) (OpenWHO, 2020; Lim et al., 2016; Shang et al., 2020; Yuki et al., 2020; Mason, 2020; Fehr et al., 2015; Abbas et al., 2004).

2.4.4 Reason behind Septic Shock and Multisystem Organ Failure (MSOF)

Leaching of cellular inflammatory components into the bloodstream leads to a systemic inflammatory response that circulates to different parts of the body. This inflammation of the lungs leads to systemic inflammatory response syndrome (SIRS). Since this systemic inflammatory response is a result of viral infection, this condition is termed as sepsis. The spread of inflammation throughout the circulatory system causes increased capillary permeability within systemic circulation. Leaking and accumulation of fluid in tissue spaces decrease overall blood volume, which results in vasodilation and in turn leads to a decrease in total peripheral resistance. A decrease in total peripheral resistance leads to a decrease in blood volume resulting in lowering the blood pressure (hypotension). This state of hypotension decreases the flow of blood to multiple organs and causes septic shock, which ultimately results in multisystem organ failure (MSOF) (OpenWHO, 2020; Lim et al., 2016; Shang et al., 2020; Yuki et al., 2020; Mason, 2020; Fehr et al., 2015; Abbas et al., 2004).

REFERENCES

Abbas, A.K., Aster, J.C., and Kumar, V. *Robbins and Cotran Pathologic Basis of Disease*, 7th ed. Philadelphia, PA: Elsevier Saunders, 2004.

Astuti, I., and Ysrafil, Y. (2020). "Severe acute respiratory syndrome coronavirus 2 (SARS-CoV-2): An overview of viral structure and host response." *Diabetes & Metabolic Syndrome*, 14 (4): 407–412. Advance online publication. Doi: 10.1016/j.dsx.2020.04.020.

Chan, J.F.-W., Kok, K.-H., Zhu, Z., Chu, H., To, K.K.-W., Yuan, S., and Yuen, K.-Y. (2020). "Genomic characterization of the 2019 novel human-pathogenic coronavirus isolated from a patient with atypical pneumonia after visiting Wuhan." *Emerging Microbes & Infections*, 9 (1): 221–236. DOI: 10.1080/22221751.2020.1719902.

Dimmock, N.J., Easton, A.J., and Leppard, K.N. (2007). *Introduction to Modern Virology*, 6th ed. Blackwell Publishing Ltd.

Fehr, A.R., and Perlman, S. (2015). "Coronaviruses: an overview of their replication and pathogenesis." *Methods in Molecular Biology (Clifton, NJ)*, 1282: 1–23. DOI: 10.1007/978-1-4939-2438-7_1.

Lim, Y.X., Ng, Y.L., Tam, J.P., and Liu, D.X. (2016). "Human coronaviruses: a review of virus-host interactions." *Diseases (Basel, Switzerland)*, 4 (3): 26. DOI: 10.3390/diseases4030026.

Mason, R.J. (2020). "Pathogenesis of COVID-19 from a cell biology perspective." *European Respiratory Journal,* 55 (4): 2000607. DOI:10.1183/13993003.00607-2020.

Neuman, B.W., Kiss, G., Kunding, A.H., Bhella, D., Baksh, M.F., Connelly, S., Droese, B., Klaus, J.P., Makino, S., Sawicki, S.G., Siddell, S.G., Stamou, D.G., Wilson, I.A., Kuhn, P., and Buchmeier, M.J. (2011). "A structural analysis of M protein in coronavirus assembly and morphology." *Journal of Structural Biology*, 174 (1): 11–22. DOI: 10.1016/j.jsb.2010.11.021.

Shang, J., Wan, Y., Luo, C., Ye, G., Geng, Q., Auerbach, A., and Li, F. (2020, May). "Cell entry mechanisms of SARS-CoV-2." *Proceedings of the National Academy of Sciences*, 117 (21): 11727–11734. DOI: 10.1073/pnas.2003138117.

Swiss Institute of Bioinformatics. Retrieved June 10, 2020, from https://viralzone.expasy.org/764?outline=all_by_species.

UniProtKB P59594. Retrieved June 10, 2020, from https://www.uniprot.org/uniprot/P59594.

UniProtKB P59595. Retrieved June 10, 2020, from https://www.uniprot.org/uniprot/P59595.

UniProtKB P59596. Retrieved June 10, 2020, from https://www.uniprot.org/uniprot/P59596.

UniProtKB P59637. Retrieved June 10, 2020, from https://www.uniprot.org/uniprot/P59637.

WHO Clinical Care Severe Acute Respiratory Illness (SARI) Training. World Health Organization. (2020). Retrieved June 22, 2020, from https://openwho.org/courses/severe-acute-respiratory-infection.

Yuki, K., Fujiogi, M., and Koutsogiannaki, S. (2020). "COVID-19 pathophysiology: a review." *Clinical Immunology (Orlando, Fla.)*, 215: 108427. DOI: 10.1016/j.clim.2020.108427.

Epidemiology, Pharmacology, Diagnosis, and Treatment of COVID-19

3

3.1 INTRODUCTION

COVID-19, in general, is a new disease. The scientific community has been studying human coronaviruses for a long time, but the outcome of exposure to novel coronavirus, SARS-CoV-2, and the disease it causes are different compared to SARS-CoV and MERS-CoV, etc. There are a number of different viruses (e.g., rhinoviruses, coronaviruses, etc.) that appear every year and cause flu symptoms in humans. For years, the same family of viruses has been appearing but with increased virulence in the subsequent year. The mutations they acquire over the years are the reason for their virulence property. The human immune system has the ability to generate immunologic memory. If a pathogen (virus) has infected an individual, the immune system develops a protective response and a memory response directed against that pathogen. The previous exposure to a certain pathogen (virus) produces immunologic memory, which is present in the form of antibodies that are designed to recognize and neutralize the specific pathogen. When the virulent form of the same pathogen infects the previously exposed individual, the components of immunologic memory take over and eliminate the threat before the symptoms get manifested. Thus the previous exposure to a pathogen provides

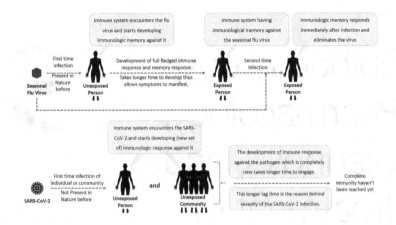

FIGURE 3.1   Seasonal flu virus and SARS-CoV-2 – comparing the intensity of infection.

human beings with a certain extent of protection. SARS-CoV-2, in contrast, has not been around in the environment previously, and hence human beings are not habituated with the virus. So when an individual comes in contact with SARS-CoV-2, the immune system recognizes it as a completely new threat and mounts a completely new set of immune responses. The development of immune response against this new pathogen takes a long time to get involved. This longer lag time is the reason behind the severity of the SARS-CoV-2 infection. Since the human body has to create a completely new set of immune memory response, the virus gets enough time and better opportunity to manifest itself and thus giving rise to the symptoms that are observable (see Figure 3.1). So, if the virus is relatively new to the human population, then the outcome of that infection will be severe compared to the infections caused by the viruses that appear annually. New virus (SARS-CoV-2) has serious symptomatology because the immune system is modifying itself to protect the system against the virus as well as to develop immunological memory against it (Lipton, 2020). This section discusses the epidemiology, pharmacology, diagnosis, and investigational treatments of COVID-19 that are currently under clinical trials.

3.2 EPIDEMIOLOGY OF COVID-19

Epidemiology is the study of distribution and determinants of health-related states or events in specified populations and the application of this study to control health problems (Dictionary of Epidemiology, 2001). The word "Epidemiology" can be divided into three parts: the first one is "epi," which in Greek means "upon;" the second part is "demos," which in Greek means "people;" and the third part is "logos," which in Greek means "to study." Epidemiology is also described as the basic science of public health. Distribution, frequency, and pattern of health events in a population are the critical aspects of epidemiology (CDC, 2020).

- **Frequency** – It refers to the number of health events (e.g., number of cases of COVID-19 in a population) as well as the relationship of that size to the total number of population. The result of such comparison (resulting rate) helps the scientists to perform a comparative study of the disease across the population (CDC, 2020).
- **Pattern** – It refers to the occurrence of health-related events based on time, place, and person. Time patterns may be seasonal, annual, hourly, weekly, daily, etc. Geographic aspects fall under the place pattern, and demographic factors, age, sex, and socioeconomic status come under the person pattern (CDC, 2020).
- **Determinants** – These may be considered as the causes and other factors that influence the occurrence of disease and other health-related events (CDC, 2020).

Knowledge of epidemiology is essential for decision making regarding the public health. It helps in the development and evaluation of interventions that are applied to the prevention and control of health-related issues. If conducted properly, epidemiology becomes a valuable asset for determining the cause of disease and for planning specific interventions.

3.2.1 Case Fatality Rate

Case fatality rate (CFR) is an important aspect that one needs to consider while analyzing the epidemiology of a particular disease. In epidemiology, CFR refers to the section of people who die due to a particular disease among all people diagnosed with the disease over a certain time period (Harrington, 2020). The general formula to calculate CFR is as follows:

$$CFR = \frac{Total\ number\ of\ deaths\ due\ to\ disease}{Total\ number\ of\ cases\ of\ the\ disease} \times 100$$

For example, the CFR of severe acute respiratory syndrome during 2002–2004 (CDC, 2004) is as follows:

$$\text{CFR (SARS: 2002}-2004)=\frac{774}{8096}\times100$$

So, the CFR (SARS 2002–2004) is 9.5%.

Similarly, the CFR of Middle East respiratory syndrome during 2012–2019 (WHO, 2019) is as follows:

$$\text{CFR (MERS: 2012}-2019)=\frac{858}{2494}\times100$$

So, the CFR (MERS 2012–2019) is 34.4%.

The CFR of COVID-19 of 2019, which is still active (WHO, 2020), is as follows:

$$\text{CFR (COVID -19: 2019}-\text{still active})=\frac{509,779}{10,434,835}\times100$$

So, the CFR (COVID-19 as of June 30, 2020) is 4.88%.

So the CFR of COVID-19 is less than that of SARS and MERS (Figures 3.2 and 3.3).

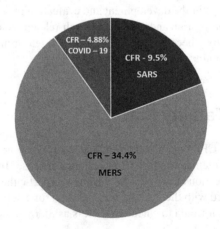

■ CFR (SARS 2002 – 2004)   ■ CFR (MERS 2012 – 2019)   ■ CFR (COVID 19 as of June 30, 2020)

FIGURE 3.2   Comparison of case fatality rate of SARS, MERS, and COVID-19.

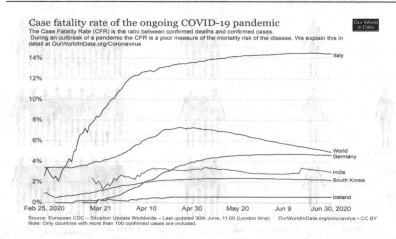

FIGURE 3.3   Case fatality rate of ongoing COVID-19 pandemic as of 30 June 2020. (European CDC: Situation Update, 2020.)

3.2.2 Basic Reproduction Number (R_0)

Similar to CFR, the concept of R-Naught (R_0) is significant in understanding the epidemiology of disease under consideration. The R_0 stands for the basic repro-duction number, which explains the degree of spreadability of any disease. For example, by considering R_0, the epidemiologists can predict how many persons one individual can infect. Let's consider that Patient 1 (P1) is suffering from COVID-19. The P1 can spread the infection to other individuals through the respiratory droplets. Researchers have reported that one COVID-19 patient (P1) can potentially spread the disease to two to three individuals. This makes the R_0 for COVID-19 to be between 2 and 3. Let's consider the worst-case scenario, that is, one person (P1) can spread the disease to three other people. Each of these three people transmits the disease to three other people, thus giving rise to nine COVID-19 patients. These nine patients give rise to 27 COVID-19 patients, and the transmission continues following the same pattern (see Figure 3.4). From the scenario, it is clear that COVID-19 cases increase exponentially. In Figure 3.5, the upward rising curve represents (R_0 COVID-19) the exponential rise of COVID-19. In comparison, the R_0 for influenza (see Table 3.1) is approximately around 1.3 (for convenience, the value is rounded to 1), which means one person has the ability to infect one other person. So, P1 infected with influenza can pass it on to the next person and so on. From the scenario, it is clear that influenza cases follow a steady growth pattern. In Figure 3.5, the flat curve represents (R_0 influenza) steady progress of influenza. Thus comparison of transmission rate indicates that COVID-19 has larger spreadability compared to influenza.

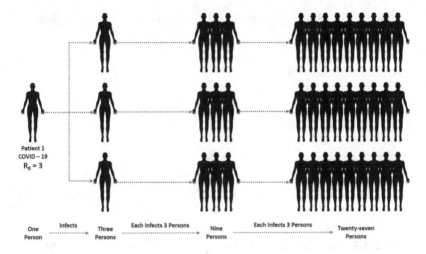

FIGURE 3.4 Degree of spreadability of COVID-19 (R_0).

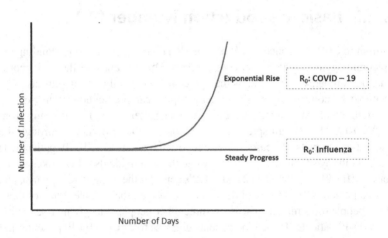

FIGURE 3.5 General curve showing R_0 of COVID-19 and influenza.

TABLE 3.1 Reproductive number of some viral diseases

Reproductive ratio (R_0): degree of spreadability

COVID-19	SARS	MERS	SEASONAL INFLUENZA
R_0: 2–3	R_0: 3–5	R_0: <1	R_0: 1–1.3

3.2.3 Serial Interval

Serial interval (SI for COVID-19) is defined as the time duration between the infector (P1) having the symptom onset and the infectee (P2) having the symptom onset (Cowling and Leung, 2020). Understanding SIs (in relation to COVID-19) is essential for determining the basic reproduction number (R_0) and the extent of interventions required to control the epidemic (Svensson, 2007). Let's understand this concept with the help of an example. Suppose P1/infector gets infected on Day 0 and develops symptoms from Day X all the way until Day 14. On the 14th day, the symptoms of P1 stop. Somewhere during the period of infection, P1/infector spreads SARS-CoV-2 to another person, P2/infectee. The P2 after coming in contact with P1 becomes infected (Day 0) and subsequently after a certain period develops the first symptom (on Day X), progresses till 14th day and then stops. Similarly during the period of infection, Patient 2 (in this case, P2 becomes the infector) and transmits the disease to Patient 3 (P3/infectee) and the progression of the disease continues in the same pattern (see Figure 3.6). The time duration from the point of onset of symptoms in P1 (Day X, P1) to the point of onset of symptoms in P2 (Day X, P2) is considered as SI (see Figure 3.6). The shorter the SI, the more fatal the virus is. The larger the value of the SI, the less risky it is. The SI for COVID-19 is approximately 5–7.5. The SI for seasonal influenza is approximately 2.5. That means the time of onset of symptoms in P1 to the point of onset of symptoms of P2 is a period of 7.5 days, whereas in the case of influenza, it is 2.5 days. So for one COVID-19, patients take approximately 7.5 days to infect the other three persons. Thus COVID-19 spreads out over

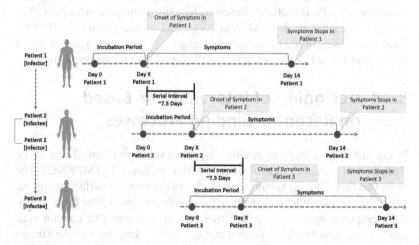

FIGURE 3.6 Concept of serial interval – COVID-19.

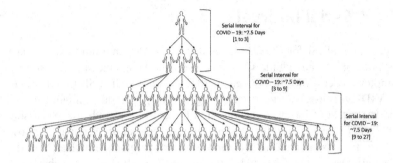

FIGURE 3.7   Serial interval and exponential rise of COVID-19 cases.

a longer period compared to the seasonal influenza (2.5 days approximately). Figure 3.7 represents the connection between the SI and the exponential rise in COVID-19 infection over a specified time period.

There is still a need for extensive understanding of COVID-19, especially the factors relating to mortality and its ability to be transmitted on a pandemic level (Petrosillo et al., 2020).

3.3 PHARMACOLOGY OF COVID-19

The present outbreak of coronavirus-associated acute respiratory disease is the third documented spillover of animal coronavirus to humans resulting in a major pandemic (WHO, 2020). Human-to-human transmission of SARS-CoV-2 occurs via respiratory droplets from cough and sneeze (WHO, 2020). This section discusses, in brief, the emerging targets for pharmacological-antiviral interventions based on various stages of the lifecycle of the coronaviruses.

3.3.1 Designing of Interventions Based on Receptor-Binding Processes

In the first step of receptor binding, S-protein is cleaved into S1 and S2 by the host cell protease, transmembrane serine protease 2 (TMPRSS2). The main function of the S1 subunit is to bind with the host cell surface receptors, while the function of S2 is to mediate the membrane fusion. One of the potential therapeutic approaches is to either develop vaccines that contain antigen derived from the spike protein that can boost recognition of the viruses by immune cells or develop monoclonal antibodies that bind to S-protein of coronaviruses and block the interaction with human cells.

TMPRSS2 can be considered as another potential therapeutic target because this structure presents on the host cell membrane is essential for the entry and spread of coronaviruses (Hoffmann et al., 2020). One chemical agent that is currently being tested on the mouse models called camostat mesylate has shown to check the spread and pathogenesis of SARS-CoV by inhibiting the TMPRSS2 activity, which is being considered as a potential candidate (Uno, 2020). Clinical trials are in progress to validate the hypothesis that camostat mesylate may be able to inhibit the SARS-CoV-2 replication in vitro. The goal of the clinical trial is to determine whether camostat mesylate decreases the viral load (SARS-CoV-2) early in COVID-19 infection (NCT04353284, 2020).

Based on the protein modeling studies, it was observed that spike protein of that SARS-CoV family has a strong binding affinity for human Angiotensin Converting Enzyme-2 [ACE-2] receptors and uses them as a mechanism for cell entry (Zhang et al., 2005). ACE-2 receptors are highly expressed in Type II alveolar cells, which are found in the lungs. However, ACE-2 receptors are also found in the heart, kidney, blood vessels, liver, and small intestine. Thus another potential drug target would be an interaction site between ACE-2 and spike protein. The compound that has recently been found in a computational study that is predicted to bind with the interface of spike–ACE-2 complex is a natural flavonoid called Hesperidin (Basu et al., 2020).

Studies in mice demonstrated that the binding of S-protein (SARS-CoV-2) to ACE-2 (host cell) leads to the downregulation of the ACE-2 receptor and thereby contributes to severe lung injury (Kuba et al., 2005). This suggests that the delivery of an excessive soluble form of ACE-2 may comparatively bind with SARS-CoV-2 and not only neutralize the virus but also rescue cellular ACE-2, which regulates the renin–angiotensin–aldosterone system to protect the lungs from injury. Various independent studies have already found recombinant human ACE-2 to be safe with no negative hemodynamic effects in healthy subjects (Zhang et al., 2020; Haschke et al., 2013; Khan et al., 2017; Zhang et al., 2017).

3.3.2 Designing of Interventions Based on Uncoating, Replication, and Translation of Viral Genetic Material

After uncoating, the genomic RNA of coronaviruses act as mRNA for translation of replicase polyproteins 1a and 1ab. Proteolytic cleavage of these polyproteins produces a number of nonstructural proteins including RNA-dependent RNA polymerase (RdRp), helicase, and nonstructural proteins 3, 4, and 6. These nonstructural proteins 3, 4, and 6 are thought to be responsible for anchoring the coronavirus replication transcription complex through recruitment of intracellular endoplasmic reticulum membranes to form double-membrane vesicles abbreviated as DMVs. RdRp and helicase localize to double-membrane vesicles and drive the production of subgenomic mRNAs from which the structural accessory protein is produced in the next phase of translation. Now RdRp is a target for investigational drugs such as remdesivir (Al-Tawfiq et al., 2020) and favipiravir (Qingxian et al., 2020). Preliminary research has shown that both of these agents inhibit RdRp and thus might be useful in the treatment of early and mid-stages of coronavirus disease.

3.3.3 Designing of Interventions Based on the Synthesis of Structural Proteins and Assembly of Viral Particles

Considering the next step of the viral lifecycle, synthesis of transmembrane structural proteins S, M, and E is inserted and folded into the Endoplasmic Reticulum (ER) and then transported to Endoplasmic Reticulum Golgi Intermediate Compartment (ERGIC). The M protein regulates the entire assembly process (Lim et al., 2016). Once the final virion assembly occurs in the intermediate compartment, mature virions are released into smooth vesicles, which then leave the cell by exocytosis. Now in addition to the investigational agents that were discussed so far, there are few antiviral drugs that are already on the market that are reported as potentially effective against coronaviruses. One of them is antimalarial drugs called chloroquine or hydroxychloroquine, which exerts its antiviral activity in part by increasing the pH in the host cell lysosomes that in turn inhibit the hydrolytic activity of protease enzymes that are required for the processing of viral glycoprotein during infection. Other drugs of interest are a combination of lopinavir-ritonavir (Cao et al., 2020) as well as darunavir-cobicistat (Chen et al., 2020), which belongs to the class of drugs known as the protease inhibitors. These drugs were originally developed to block HIV replication. However, molecular docking studies have shown that they may also interact with some protein that is required for the replication of coronavirus (Odhar et al., 2020).

3.4 DIAGNOSIS OF COVID-19

Diagnosis can be considered as an art of identifying a disease from its signs and symptoms (Merriam-Webster, n.d.). A sign is the outcome of a disease condition that can be observed by someone else, for example, coughing, sneezing, and rise in body temperature, whereas symptoms are the effects experienced only by the person who has the condition, for example, headache, the feeling of tightness in the chest, muscular pain, and severe weakness. It takes around 5–6 days for symptoms to manifest.

According to the World Health Organization as updated till June 30, 2020, the cases of COVID-19 are identified by two methods:

1. Serology-based diagnostic tests
2. Real-time reverse transcriptase-polymerase chain reaction (RT-PCR)

Serology-based tests (detects immune response to SARS-CoV-2 exposure) – These are blood tests that are used to detect whether a person is infected with SARS-CoV-2 or not by analyzing specific products of the immune response. In medicine, serology means the scientific study of serum, and in general practice, it refers to the diagnostic identification of antibodies in serum. A significant aspect that one needs to understand is that these tests do not directly detect SARS-CoV-2 in the patient's body, but just detects the presence or absence of antibodies specific for SARS-CoV-2. The positive test result implies that the person's immune system has developed antibodies against SARS-CoV-2, which helps in knowing that the person was infected by the pathogen. Serological tests are used to screen individuals who are asymptomatic or have recovered. Table 3.2 provides a brief idea about the types of serological assays.

RT-PCR Test (detects active SARS-CoV-2 infection) – The RT-PCR is being implemented globally for diagnosing COVID-19 cases. This test identifies viruses based on their genetic fingerprint. RT-PCR can only indicate the

TABLE 3.2   Types of serological tests for COVID-19

Types of serological diagnostic tests

Rapid diagnostic tests (RDTs) for COVID-19

- **Sample Needed:** Blood samples obtained by finger pricking, saliva, nasal swab fluids.
- **Time Required for the Test:** 10–30 minutes (approximately).
- **Advantages:** It detects the presence or absence of antibodies against SARS-CoV-2 in a patient's serum. This is a portable test.
- **Disadvantages:** It does not detect the amount of antibodies present in the patient' serum.It does not provide any information whether these antibodies are able to inhibit the growth of the virus.

(Continued)

TABLE 3.2 (*Continued*) Types of serological tests for COVID-19

Types of serological diagnostic tests

Enzyme-linked immunosorbent assay (ELISA) for COVID-19
- **Sample Needed:** Whole blood, plasma, or serum.
- **Time Required for the Test:** 2–5 hours.
- **Advantages:** It detects the presence or absence of antibodies against SARS-CoV-2 in a patient's serum. This is a laboratory-based test. It detects the amount of antibody present in the patient' serum.
- **Disadvantages:** It does not provide any information whether those antibodies are able to inhibit the growth of the virus.

Neutralization assay for COVID-19
- **Sample Needed:** Whole blood, plasma, or serum.
- **Time Required for the Test:** 3–5 days.
- **Advantages:** The presence of active antibodies in patient serum that are able to inhibit SARS-CoV-2 growth cell culture system. This is a laboratory based test.
- **Disadvantages:** It may miss antibodies to viral proteins that are not involved in replication.

Chemiluminescent immunoassay for COVID-19
- **Sample Needed:** Whole blood, plasma, serum.
- **Time Required for the Test:** 1–2 hours.
- **Advantages:** It detects the presence or absence of antibodies against SARS-CoV-2 in a patient's serum. This is a laboratory-based test.
- **Disadvantages:** It does not provide any information whether those antibodies are able to inhibit growth of the virus.

presence of viral genetic material during infection. This test does not specify whether the person was infected and subsequently recovered.

The steps involved during RT-PCR for COVID-19:

- Collection of specimen (of suspected COVID-19 case).
- Extraction of RNA from the specimen.
- Conversion of extracted RNA into complementary DNA.
- Amplification of complementary DNA by PCR with SARS-CoV-2-specific primers.
- Interpretation of the results.

The series of steps involved in the diagnosis of COVID-19 using RT-PCR is shown schematically in Figure 3.8.

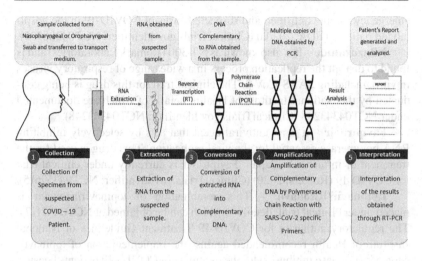

FIGURE 3.8 Basic steps involved in RT-PCR analysis of COVID-19.

3.5 CONVENTIONAL TREATMENT OF COVID-19

Based on the reports published by the World Health Organization on their official website as of 30 June 2020, there are no specific vaccines or medicines available for COVID-19 (WHO, 2020). Supportive care may be provided to infected patients in order to alleviate the symptoms. In severe cases, supportive care to the vital organs is advised (CDC, 2020). This section discusses in brief the various experimental drugs that are presently under clinical trials and their implementation status. It is to be understood that all the following therapeutic agents are under clinical trial, and the details regarding the outcome may change in the future.

3.5.1 Investigational Antiviral Agents

Remdesivir – It is considered as a broad-spectrum antiviral agent, also known as GS-5734 (Gilead Sciences, Inc.) (FDA, 2020c). Chemically, it is a nucleotide analog prodrug, which means the chemical that mimics the actual nucleotide molecule. Remdesivir was approved by the FDA (United States) per the guidelines of Emergency Use Authorization (EUA) on 1 May 2020 for emergency use in confirmed and suspected cases of COVID-19 in the hospitalized patients (FDA, 2020a) (ClinicalTrials.gov Identifier: NCT04280705).

Nitazoxanide – It is also known as NT-300 (Romark Laboratories) and is found to disrupt the replication process in a wide range of respiratory viruses in vitro, including SARS-CoV-2. The clinical trial for this drug is being conducted by the National Institute of Health, details of which are documented under NCT04343248 (ClinicalTrials.gov Identifier: NCT04343248).

Favipiravir – It is an antiviral agent that acts by selectively inhibiting RNA polymerase essential for the viral replication. This drug is used for the treatment of influenza in Japan. Favipiravir is currently under clinical trial for COVID-19 (Reuters, 2020) (ClinicalTrials.gov Identifier: NCT04359615).

Lopinavir/Ritonavir – This combination of lopinavir/ritonavir is placed under clinical trial, details of which can be obtained at NCT04321174. The regulatory authority for COVID-19 Treatment Guidelines of National Institute of Health recommended against the implementation of lopinavir/ritonavir (protease inhibitors) for the treatment of COVID-19 patients because it did not show significant benefit in patients with COVID-19 (NIH, 2020c) (ClinicalTrials.gov Identifier: NCT04321174).

Chloroquine or Hydroxychloroquine – Effectivity of chloroquine in inhibiting SARS-CoV-2 in vitro was reported by Wang et al. (2020). Food and Drug Association (FDA, United States) revoked the Emergency Use Authorization (EUA) for hydroxychloroquine and chloroquine on 15 June 2020 (FDA, 2020b). During the clinical trial, the drug was found to be ineffective in treating COVID-19 in hospitalized patients and shown to create adverse drug reactions.

3.5.2 Immunomodulators and Other Investigational Therapies

Interleukin-6 Inhibitors – Interleukin 6 (IL-6) is a pleiotropic (producing more than one effect), proinflammatory (promotes inflammation) cytokine produced by various cells involved in the immune response. SARS-CoV-2 infection induces the production of IL-6 from bronchial epithelial cells. This series of events is the reason for considering IL-6 inhibitors as potential therapeutic agents. As of 11 June 2020, the National Institutes of Health reported that there is insufficient data to recommend for or against the use of IL-6 inhibitors (NIH, 2020a).

Interleukin-1 Inhibitors – The COVID-19 patients have been found to have elevated levels of Interleukin 1 (IL-1). IL-1 inhibitors have been implemented for treating elevated levels of IL-1 in COVID-19 patients, but it did not show any significant outcome. On 11 June 2020, the National Institutes of Health reported that there are insufficient data to recommend either for or against the use of IL-1 inhibitors for the treatment of COVID-19 (NIH, 2020b).

Convalescent Plasma – Convalescent plasma is antibody-rich plasma (antibodies specific for SARS-CoV-2) obtained from individuals (eligible donors) who have recovered from COVID-19. The plasma therapy has not yet shown promising clinical outcomes in treating patients with COVID-19. The Food and Drug Administration (FDA, United States) recommended a thorough investigation for the determination of safety and efficacy through regulated clinical trials before declaring it a therapy for COVID-19. On 1 May 2020, Food and Drug Administration (FDA, United States) has released Recommendations for Investigational COVID-19 Convalescent Plasma, which provide guidelines for healthcare providers and researchers on administration and study of investigational convalescent plasma obtained from individual who has recovered from COVID-19 (FDA, 2020d). Convalescent plasma therapy has not yet been approved for use by FDA and is currently being regulated as an investigational procedure (FDA, 2020d) (Figure 3.9).

Corticosteroids – The World Health Organization released interim guidance on 27 May 2020 on Clinical Management of COVID-19 in which they recommended against the routine use of systemic corticosteroids for the treatment of viral pneumonia (WHO, 2020). Russell et al. reported that corticosteroids produce immunosuppressive effects that may lead to adverse reactions and have failed to provide a significant benefit over other viral epidemics such as SARS and MERS (Russell, et al. 2020) (Figure 3.10).

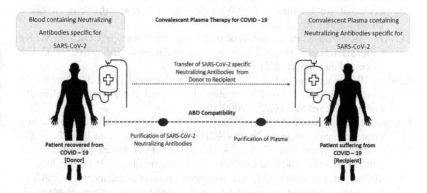

FIGURE 3.9 Convalescent plasma therapy for COVID-19.

Treatment Highlights as of June 30, 2020 based on reports published by

World Health Organization

✓ No specific Medicines or Vaccines are available for COVID – 19.

✓ Research and Clinical Trials are in progress worldwide.

✓ Optimized supportive care delivery is recommended.

✓ Early recognition of High Risk groups and Access to Critical Care Interventions are necessary.

✓ Diagnosis and Treatment of co-infections and other endemic diseases are important.

FIGURE 3.10 Highlights of treatment for COVID-19 as of June 2020. (www. who.int.)

REFERENCES

Al-Tawfiq, J.A., Al-Homoud, A.H., and Memish, Z.A. (2020). "Remdesivir as a possible therapeutic option for the COVID-19." *Travel Medicine and Infectious Disease*, 34: 101615. DOI: 10.1016/j.tmaid.2020.101615.

Basu, A., Sarkar, A., and Maulik, U. (2020). "Computational approach for the design of potential spike protein binding natural compounds in SARS - CoV2." DOI:10.21203/rs.3.rs-33181/v1.

Cao, B., Wang, Y., Wen, D., et al. (2020). "A trial of Lopinavir–Ritonavir in Covid-19." *The New England Journal of Medicine*, 382 (21). DOI:10.1056/nejmc2008043.

Chen, J., Xia, L., Liu, L., et al. (2020). "Antiviral activity and safety of darunavir/cobicistat for treatment of COVID-19." *Open Forum Infectious Diseases*. DOI:10.1093/ofid/ofaa241.

COVID-19 Ring-Based Prevention Trial with Lopinavir/Ritonavir (CORIPREV-LR). ClinicalTrials.gov. Available at https://clinicaltrials.gov/ct2/show/NCT04321174. Accessed on June 22, 2020.

Cowling, B.J., and Leung, G.M. (2020). "Epidemiological research priorities for public health control of the ongoing global novel coronavirus (2019-nCoV) outbreak." *Euro Surveill*, 25: 2000110.

Favipiravir in Hospitalized COVID-19 Patients (FIC). ClinicalTrials.gov. Available at https://clinicaltrials.gov/ct2/show/NCT04359615. Accessed on June 22, 2020.

FDA. (2020a). Coronavirus (COVID – 19) Update: FDA Issues Emergency Use Authorization for Potential COVID – 19 Treatment. fda.gov. Retrieved June 22, 2020, from https://www.fda.gov/news-events/press-announcements/coronavirus-covid-19-update-fda-issues-emergency-use-authorization-potential-covid-19-treatment.

FDA. (2020b). Coronavirus (COVID-19) Update: FDA Revokes Emergency Use Authorization for Chloroquine and Hydroxychloroquine. U.S. Food and Drug Administration. Available at: https://www.fda.gov/news-events/press-announcements/coronavirus-covid-19-update-fda-revokes-emergency-use-authorization-chloroquine-and. June 15, 2020.

FDA. (2020c, June). Factsheet for Healthcare Providers Emergency Use Authorization (EUA) of Remdesivir (GS-5734™). fda.gov. Retrieved from https://www.fda.gov/media/137566/download. Revised on June 22, 2020.

FDA. (2020d, May 1). Recommendations for Investigational COVID – 19 Convalescent Plasma [Guideline]. Available at https://www.fda.gov/vaccines-blood-biologics/investigational-new-drug-ind-or-device-exemption-ide-process-cber/recommendations-investigational-covid-19-convalescent-plasma. Accessed on June 22, 2020.

Fujifilm to Start Phase II Clinical Trial of Avigan for COVID-19 Patients in U.S. Reuters. Available at https://www.reuters.com/article/us-health-coronavirus-fujifilm-avigan/fujifilm-to-start-phase-ii-clinical-trial-of-avigan-for-covid-19-patients-in-u-s-idUSKCN21R0KF. April 8, 2020.

Haschke, M., Schuster, M., Poglitsch, M., Loibner, H., Salzberg, M., Bruggisser, M., Penninger, J., and Krahenbuhl, S. (2013) "Pharmacokinetics and pharmaco-dynamics of recombinant human angiotensin-converting enzyme 2 in healthy human subjects." *Clinical Pharmacokinetics*, 52: 783–792.

Hoffmann, M., Kleine-Weber, H., Schroeder, S., et al. (2020). "SARS-CoV-2 cell entry depends on ACE2 and TMPRSS2 and is blocked by a clinically proven protease inhibitor." *Cell*, 181: 1–10. DOI: 10.1016/j.cell.2020.02.052.

Khan A., Benthin C., Zeno B., et al. (2017). "A pilot clinical trial of recombinant human angiotensin-converting enzyme 2 in acute respiratory distress syndrome." *Critical Care*, 21: 234.

Kuba, K., Imai, Y., Rao, S., et al. (2005). "A crucial role of angiotensin converting enzyme 2 (ACE2) in SARS coronavirus-induced lung injury." *Nature Medicine*, 11 (8): 875–879. DOI: 10.1038/nm1267.

Last J.M., editor. (2001). *Dictionary of Epidemiology*, 4th ed. New York: Oxford University Press, 61.

Lim, Y.X., Ng, Y.L., Tam, J.P., and Liu, D.X. (2016). "Human coronaviruses: a review of virus-host interactions." *Diseases (Basel, Switzerland)*, 4 (3): 26. DOI: 10.3390/diseases4030026.

Merriam-Webster. (n.d.). Diagnosis. In *Merriam-Webster.com dictionary*. Retrieved June 23, 2020, from https://www.merriam-webster.com/dictionary/diagnosis.

Lipton, B. H., PhD (2020, March 30). Bruce Lipton on COVID-19, Coronavirus Pandemic & Evolution [Video] Available at https://www.youtube.com/watch?v=oyijHfL-W7w&t=2728s/. Accessed on June 27, 2020.

NIH. (2020a). Interleukin-6 Inhibitors, COVID – 19 Treatment Guidelines [Guideline]. Available at https://www.covid19treatmentguidelines.nih.gov/immune-based-therapy/interleukin-6-inhibitors/. Accessed on June 22, 2020.

NIH. (2020b). Interleukin-1 Inhibitors, COVID – 19 Treatment Guidelines [Guideline]. Available at https://www.covid19treatmentguidelines.nih.gov/immune-based-therapy/interleukin-1-inhibitors/. Accessed on June 22, 2020.

NIH. (2020c). Potential Antiviral Drugs under Evaluation for the Treatment of COVID – 19. COVID – 19 Treatment Guidelines [Guideline]. Available at https://www.covid19treatmentguidelines.nih.gov/antiviral-therapy/. Accessed on June 22, 2020.

Odhar, H.A., Ahjel, S.W., Albeer, A., Hashim, A.F., Rayshan, A.M., and Humadi, S.S. (2020). "Molecular docking and dynamics simulation of FDA approved drugs with the main protease from 2019 novel coronavirus." *Bioinformation*, 16 (3): 236–244. https://doi.org/10.6026/97320630016236.

Petrosillo, N., Viceconte, G., Ergonul, O., Ippolito, G., and Petersen, E. (2020). "COVID-19, SARS and MERS: are they closely related?" *Clinical Microbiology and Infection: The Official Publication of the European Society of Clinical Microbiology and Infectious Diseases*, 26 (6): 729–734. DOI: 10.1016/j.cmi.2020.03.026.

Qingxian, C., Minghui, Y., Dongjing, L., et al. (2020). "Experimental treatment with Favipiravir for COVID – 19: an open label control study." *Engineering*, Elsevier, DOI: 10.1016/j.eng.2020.03.007 Retrieved on June 22, 2020.

Russell, C.D., Millar, J.E., and Baillie, J.K. (2020). "Clinical evidence does not support corticosteroid treatment for 2019-nCoV lung injury." *Lancet (London, England)*, 395 (10223): 473–475. DOI: 10.1016/S0140–6736(20)30317-2.

Svensson, A.A. (2007). "Note on generation times in epidemic models." *Mathematical Biosciences*, 208: 300–11.

Trial to Evaluate the Efficacy and Safety of Nitazoxanide (NTZ) for Post Exposure Prophylaxis of COVID – 19 and Other Viral Respiratory Illnesses in Elderly Residents of Long-Term Care Facilities (LTCF) ClinicalTrials.gov. Available at https://clinicaltrials.gov/ct2/show/NCT04343248?term=nitazoxanide&recrs=ab&cond=COVID&draw=2 Accessed on June 22, 2020.

Uno, Y. (2020). "Camostat Mesylate therapy for COVID-19." *Internal and Emergency Medicine*: 1–2. Advance online publication. DOI: 10.1007/s11739-020-02345-9.

Vinetz, J. (2020). Camostat Mesylate in COVID 19 Outpatients (Yale University). Identification Number. NCT04353284. Retrieved June 22, 2020, from https://clinicaltrials.gov/ct2/show/NCT04353284.

Wang, M., Cao, R., Zhang, L. et al. (2020). "Remdesivir and chloroquine effectively inhibit the recently emerged novel coronavirus (2019-nCoV) in vitro." *Cell Research*, 30: 269–271. DOI: 10.1038/s41422-020-0282-0.

WHO. (2020, May 27). Clinical Management of COVID – 19 [Guideline], Interim Guidance. Available at https://www.who.int/publications/i/item/clinical-management-of-severe-acute-respiratory-infection-when-novel-coronavirus-(ncov)-infection-is-suspected Accessed on June 22, 2020.

Zhang, H., and Baker, A. (2017). "Recombinant human ACE2: acing out angiotensin II in ARDS therapy." *Critical Care*, 21: 305.

Zhang, H., Penninger, J.M., Li, Y. et al. (2020). "Angiotensin-converting enzyme 2 (ACE2) as a SARS-CoV-2 receptor: molecular mechanisms and potential therapeutic target." *Intensive Care Medicine*, 46: 586–590. DOI: 10.1007/s00134-020-05985-9.

Zhang, Y., Zheng, N., Hao, P., Cao, Y., and Zhong, Y. (2005). "A molecular docking model of SARS-CoV S1 protein in complex with its receptor, human ACE2." *Computational Biology and Chemistry*, 29(3): 254–257. DOI: 10.1016/j.compbiolchem.2005.04.008.

COVID-19 Precautions and Management Strategies

4

4.1 INTRODUCTION

COVID-19 is a disease of the respiratory system caused by a coronavirus known as SARS-CoV-2. SARS-CoV-2 gets transmitted from an infected person to a healthy person through respiratory droplets and droplet nuclei (primary modes of transmission) mainly via coughing, sneezing, or talking (see Chapter 1, Section 1.7) (WHO, 2014). Transmission through droplets is possible when an individual is in close contact generally within 1 m with the infected person or the droplets remain in the air for a long time and get transmitted to individuals over distances greater than 1 m (WHO, 2020b). The virus can also get transmitted through the objects contaminated with infectious agents. Touching of eyes, nose, or mouth with unclean hand increases an individual's risk of getting infected. When in situations where complete information regarding the characteristics of the virus and proper treatment for the disease is not available, prevention measures are the only way of protection (for now) (WHO, 2020b). The World Health Organization has recommended various safety measures that may help prevent and control the spread of the disease specifically for the general public. This chapter discusses, in brief, some of the basic preventive measures such as respiratory etiquette, hand hygiene, physical distancing, and surface cleaning. It is essential that people must follow these safety measures to keep the spread of the disease under control.

4.2 MAINTAINING PROPER HAND HYGIENE

In general, the term "hand hygiene" means cleaning of hands. Hands can be cleaned either using alcohol-based hand sanitizers or using soap and water. The virus SARS-CoV-2 is made up of genetic material enclosed in a lipid covering that contains the spike protein. The soaps and sanitizers have the ability to breakdown the lipid covering, thus disorganizing the virus particle, which in turn fails to infect the host cells. The inactive fragments of the virus get washed away when rinsed with clean water. Further, the process of rubbing hands helps in the removal of microorganisms and dirt from hands. Figure 4.5 shows the ways by which maintaining proper hand hygiene provides protection against COVID-19. Implementation of proper hand hygiene measures as recommended by the World Health Organization can help check the spread of the disease (Gavi, 2020; WHO, 2009; OpenWHO, 2020).

- **Washing Hands with Alcohol-Based Hand Sanitizers** – This should be used in a situation where the hands are not visibly dirty. The primary advantage (among many) of washing hands with alcohol-based hand sanitizers is that it destroys microorganisms more effectively compared to soap and water. The alcohol present in the hand sanitizers destroys microorganisms by denaturing their protective outer membrane. The alcohol contained in the hand sanitizers are flammable and should be kept away from the flame. Washing hands with alcohol-based hand sanitizers has several advantages in comparison with that using soap and water (OpenWHO, 2020).
  - Hands can be sanitized in only about 20–30 seconds.
  - Hand sanitizers can be carried and used anywhere anytime.
  - Hand sanitizers can be applied directly and do not require a dedicated setup, that is, it does not require sinks, water, or towels.

The following steps recommended by the World Health Organization should be followed while washing hands with alcohol-based hand sanitizers (see Figure 4.1).

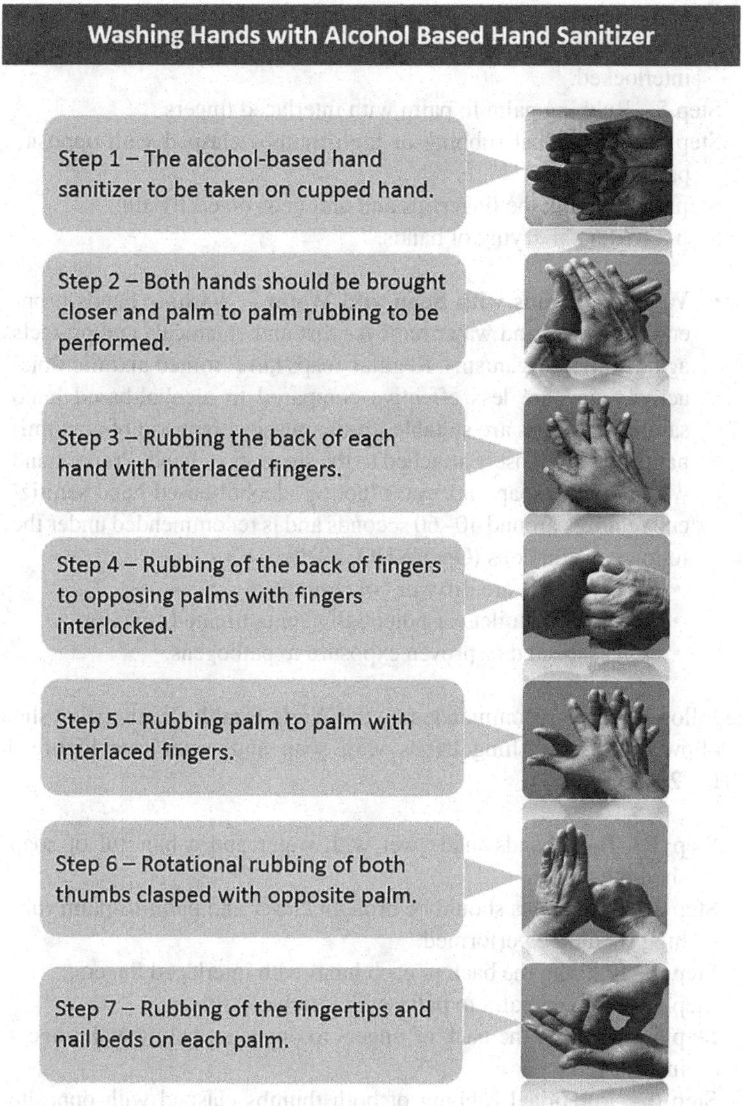

Washing Hands with Alcohol Based Hand Sanitizer

Step 1 – The alcohol-based hand sanitizer to be taken on cupped hand.

Step 2 – Both hands should be brought closer and palm to palm rubbing to be performed.

Step 3 – Rubbing the back of each hand with interlaced fingers.

Step 4 – Rubbing of the back of fingers to opposing palms with fingers interlocked.

Step 5 – Rubbing palm to palm with interlaced fingers.

Step 6 – Rotational rubbing of both thumbs clasped with opposite palm.

Step 7 – Rubbing of the fingertips and nail beds on each palm.

FIGURE 4.1 Steps of washing hands with alcohol-based hand sanitizer.

Step 1 – The alcohol-based hand sanitizer to be taken on the cupped hands.

Step 2 – Both hands should be brought closer and palm-to-palm rubbing should be performed.

Step 3 – Rubbing the back of each hand with interlaced fingers.
Step 4 – Rubbing the back of fingers to opposing palms with fingers interlocked.
Step 5 – Rubbing palm to palm with interlaced fingers.
Step 6 – Rotational rubbing of both thumbs clasped with opposite palm.
Step 7 – Rubbing the fingertips and nail beds on each palm.
Step 8 – Manual drying of hands.

- **Washing Hands with Soap and Water** – Washing hands properly with soap and water removes dirt and chemicals and protects against microorganisms. Regular soaps have limited antimicrobial activity and are less effective compared to alcohol-based hand sanitizers. Soaps are suitable for the physical removal of contaminants that are loosely attached to the surfaces of hand. Proper hand washing with soap and water (not by alcohol-based hand sanitizers) requires around 40–60 seconds and is recommended under the following situations (OpenWHO, 2020):
  - When hands are dirty or contaminated.
  - After using toilets or potentially contaminated surfaces.
  - On suspected or proven exposure to pathogens.

The following steps recommended by the World Health Organization should be followed while washing hands with soap and water (see Figure 4.2) (WHO, 2020a):

Step 1 – Both hands made wet with water and a handful of soap should be taken.
Step 2 – Both hands should be brought closer and palm-to-palm rubbing should be performed.
Step 3 – Rubbing the back of each hand with interlaced fingers.
Step 4 – Rubbing palm to palm with interlaced fingers.
Step 5 – Rubbing the back of fingers to opposing palms with fingers interlocked.
Step 6 – Rotational rubbing of both thumbs clasped with opposite palm.
Step 7 – Rubbing the fingertips and nail beds on each palm.
Step 8 – Rinsing of hands with clean water.
Step 9 – Drying of hands using disposable towels.

- **Drying of Hands after Washing** – The proper technique of drying hands is equally important as washing them. Hands that are not

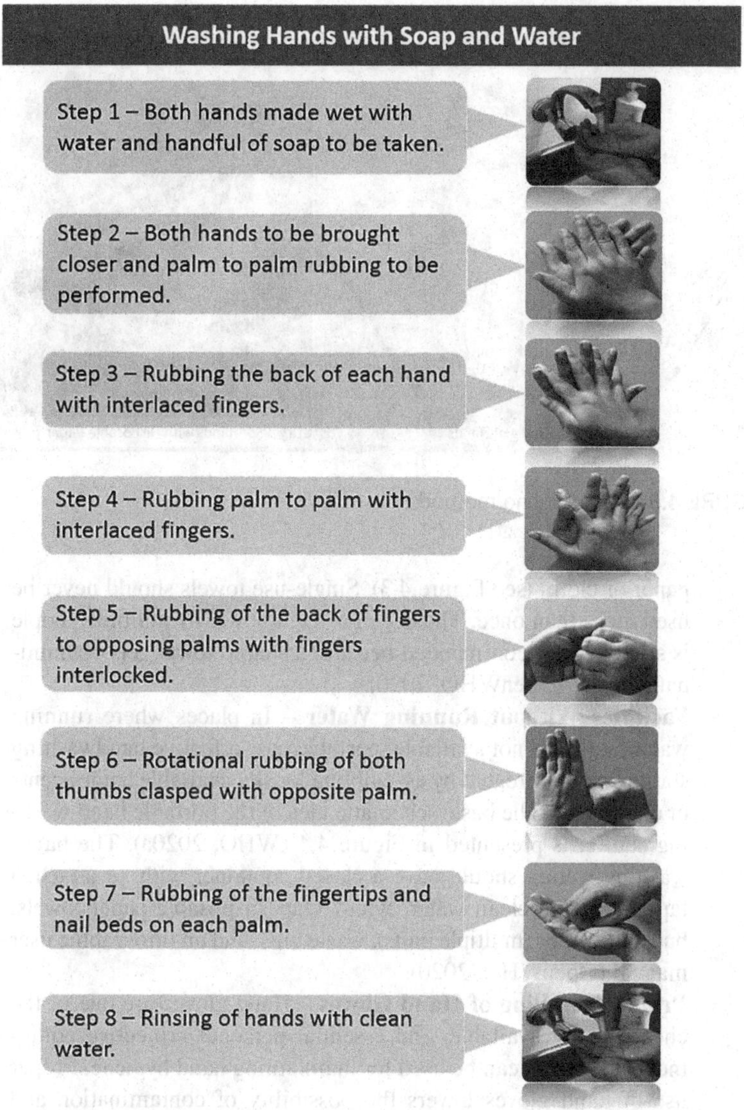

Washing Hands with Soap and Water

Step 1 – Both hands made wet with water and handful of soap to be taken.

Step 2 – Both hands to be brought closer and palm to palm rubbing to be performed.

Step 3 – Rubbing the back of each hand with interlaced fingers.

Step 4 – Rubbing palm to palm with interlaced fingers.

Step 5 – Rubbing of the back of fingers to opposing palms with fingers interlocked.

Step 6 – Rotational rubbing of both thumbs clasped with opposite palm.

Step 7 – Rubbing of the fingertips and nail beds on each palm.

Step 8 – Rinsing of hands with clean water.

FIGURE 4.2 Steps of washing hands with soap and water.

dried properly after washing hands with soap and water increase the likelihood of transmission of microorganisms through wet surfaces. Drying may be performed either by air drying (drying manually by moving hands) or using a disposable towel (made from

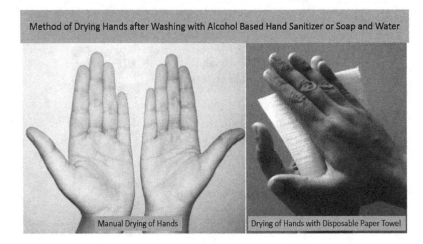

Method of Drying Hands after Washing with Alcohol Based Hand Sanitizer or Soap and Water

Manual Drying of Hands   Drying of Hands with Disposable Paper Towel

FIGURE 4.3   Hand drying methods.

paper or cloth) (see Figure 4.3). Single-use towels should never be used more than once. The use of a single towel by multiple people is strictly not recommended because a shared towel gets contaminated faster (OpenWHO, 2020).

- **Facilities Without Running Water** – In places where running water facility is not available, portable cost-effective handwashing station may be created by assembling locally available components or equipment. The basic schematic idea of the portable hand washing station is presented in Figure 4.4 (WHO, 2020a). The handwashing station should have a closed container with an attached tap containing clean water, liquid soap, disposable paper towels, buckets or tubs (multiple units), waste bins, and an infographic user manual (OpenWHO, 2020).

- **Proper Handling of Hand Gloves** – Hand gloves are one of the cheap, easily available, and essential personal protective equipment (PPE) that can be used for maintaining hand hygiene. Proper use of hand gloves lowers the possibility of contamination and reduces the spread of pathogens. Washing of hands frequently and thoroughly with soap and water or alcohol-based hand sanitizers is mandatory even if the individual is using hand gloves (WHO, 2009). The following points must be kept in mind while using hand gloves (OpenWHO, 2020):

  - An individual may use hand gloves if there was a contact with potentially infectious materials or hazardous substances.

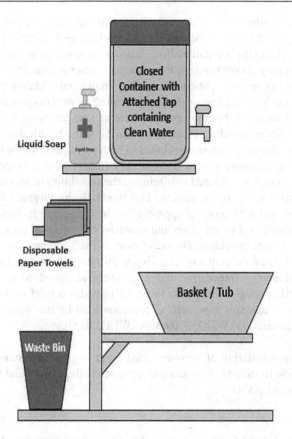

FIGURE 4.4 Schematic representation of portable hand washing station (OpenWHO, 2020).

- One should wash their hands thoroughly with soap and water or alcohol-based hand rubs before putting on hand gloves.
- Hand gloves should be removed once the desired task is complete. General nonreusable hand gloves should be disposed of properly (following safety measures) after one-time use.
- Healthcare workers or caregivers must not use the same pair of hand gloves for caring for more than one patient.
- One should again wash their hands thoroughly with soap and water or alcohol-based hand rubs after the removal of hand gloves.
- **Hand Hygiene for Individuals while Caring for Patients –** Individuals caring for patients always have an increased risk of

contracting as well as transmitting various kinds of pathogenic microorganisms. The healthcare workers and caregivers need to take extra precautions for ensuring complete hand hygiene so that they do not transmit the pathogenic microorganisms between patients or from patients to healthy individuals. Maintenance of proper hand hygiene on the part of healthcare workers prevents contamination of the environment where patients are being taken care of. While attending patients, the hands of the healthcare workers get colonized with various kinds of both pathogenic and nonpathogenic microorganisms. So it is very important that proper hand hygiene is maintained to minimize the possibility of transmission while caring for the patient. The World Health Organization has designed a "5-moment approach" of hand hygiene to prevent the transmission of infection and ensuring the safety of patients and healthcare providers. The major focus of the 5-moment approach is mainly on the contacts occurring within the patient zone (surfaces and items temporarily and exclusively allocated to a patient) while caring for patients. Table 4.1 provides a brief overview of the "5-moment approach" as recommended by the World Health Organization (WHO, 2009; OpenWHO, 2020).

Proper implementation of recommended hand hygiene measures prevents the infection from spreading and thus protects both patients and healthcare workers or caregivers.

TABLE 4.1   The World Health Organization's 5-moment approach of hand hygiene

Moment 1 – Performing hand hygiene before touching a patient
- There is always a risk for hands of healthcare workers or caregivers being contaminated with microorganisms (pathogenic and nonpathogenic).
- If proper hand hygiene is not performed before touching a patient, the caregivers may unknowingly transmit the pathogenic microorganisms to their patients.
- It is important that healthcare workers and caregivers must perform proper hand hygiene before touching a patient.
  Moment 1 ensures that microorganisms carried on the hands of healthcare workers and caregivers do not get transmitted to their patients.

(Continued)

TABLE 4.1 (*Continued*) The World Health Organization's 5-moments approach of hand hygiene

Moment 2 – Performing hand hygiene before a clean or antiseptic procedure

- Before performing antiseptic procedures, it is important to make sure that the site requiring care (critical site) does not get contaminated or exposed to microorganisms from the hand of the healthcare workers or caregivers.
- The site of the patient's body requiring antiseptic care is vulnerable to infectious agents.
- Following proper hand hygiene before performing a clean or antiseptic procedures on patients is advisable to minimize the risk.

    Moment 2 ensures that the infection with microorganisms (at the critical site) is checked while antiseptic procedures are being performed on a patient.

Moment 3 – Performing hand hygiene after exposure to body fluids

- Blood and body fluids of patients may contain infectious agents.
- Improper handling of blood and body fluids increases the risk of contamination by infectious agents and transmission of the diseases.
- Healthcare workers or caregivers must perform proper hand hygiene measures immediately after being exposed to blood or body fluids.

    Moment 3 ensures the protection of both healthcare workers or caregivers and the healthcare environment from the infectious agents present in blood and body fluids.

Moment 4 – Performing hand hygiene after touching a patient

- Coming in contact with patients increases the risk of exposure to infectious agents.
- Healthcare workers or caregivers must perform hand hygiene after touching each patient.

    Moment 4 ensures the protection of both healthcare workers or caregivers and the healthcare environment from the infectious agents present on the patient's body.

Moment 5 – Performing hand hygiene after touching the patient's surrounding

- It is known that infectious agents (like SARS-CoV-2) can get transmitted directly through fomites.
- Healthcare workers and caregivers must perform proper hand hygiene after touching any object or furniture in the patient's immediate surroundings.

    Moment 5 ensures that the infectious agent does not spread out from inside the patient zone to the rest of the surroundings.

4.3 MAINTAINING PROPER RESPIRATORY ETIQUETTE

The term "respiratory etiquette" refers to infection prevention measures to decrease the transmission of respiratory illnesses. A respiratory infection is transmitted when an infected individual sneezes or coughs and releases respiratory droplets. The droplets released from sneeze or cough can travel for several feet reaching the nose or the mouth of others. Viruses can spread easily from an infected individual to a healthy individual through direct contact via touching or shaking hands. It is not always possible to check who is infectious and who is not, because some individuals cough without having respiratory infections (e.g., patients with Chronic Obstructive Pulmonary Disease [COPD]). So maintaining proper respiratory etiquette is essential for protecting oneself from the disease (prevention) and preventing others from being exposed to the disease (source control) (Virginia Department of Health, 2011). Figure 4.5 points out the ways by which maintaining proper respiratory etiquette provides protection against COVID-19. Implementation of proper respiratory hygiene measures as recommended by the World Health Organization can help check the spread of the disease.

- **Covering the Mouth While Coughing or Sneezing** – SARS-CoV-2 present in respiratory droplets spreads through coughing, sneezing, or talking. Covering nose and mouth and sneezing into a flexed elbow is a good practice (WHO, 2020a).
- **Using Disposable Tissues or Towels** – Disposable tissues can be used while coughing or sneezing. After sneezing or coughing, the used tissues must be disposed of properly and safely preferably in a closed bin. Proper hand hygiene should be performed after disposing of the tissue (WHO, 2020a).
- **Wearing Masks (PPE)** – Masks when used along with proper respiratory etiquette and hand hygiene measures provide a general barrier that helps in lowering the infection transmission rate. The World Health Organization recommends the use of masks only as a part of a comprehensive strategy. The masks are of two basic types, medical mask and nonmedical mask (WHO, 2020a).
  - **Medical Masks** – These are also known as surgical masks and prevent individuals from spreading the infection and also protect an individual from getting infected. Healthcare workers, patients suffering from COVID-19, individuals caring for COVID-19 patients, old-aged persons (above 60 years),

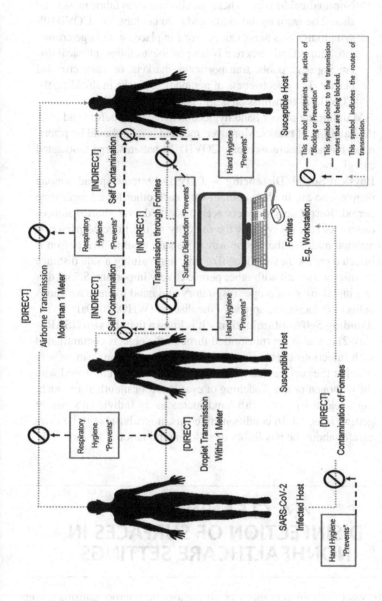

FIGURE 4.5 Schematic representation of ways by which respiratory hygiene, hand hygiene, and surface disinfection help in the prevention of COVID-19.

and individuals with underlying health conditions should use medical masks (WHO, 2020a).

- **Nonmedical Masks** – These are also known as fabric masks and should be worn by individuals who do not have any COVID-19 symptoms. This mask can be worn in places with large crowds most importantly where it is not possible to follow physical distancing (e.g., public transportation, markets, or other crowded places). The effectiveness of nonmedical masks in shielding the COVID-19 transmission is still not clear (WHO, 2020a).

Maintaining proper hand hygiene is mandatory before and after the handling of masks. Moreover, medical masks should be prioritized for healthcare workers, COVID-19 patients, and associated caregivers.

- **Physical/Social Distancing** – COVID-19 may spread among people who are in close contact with each other for a longer time period. Respiratory droplets get transmitted over short distances faster. As it is known that the majority of the infected person is asymptomatic so there is no way to be sure whether that person is infected or not. In situations like this, maintaining a safe distance (of minimum 1 m) with other people is very important. Social distancing along with proper respiratory and hand hygiene measures helps in reducing the spread of the disease (WHO, 2020a).

- **Avoiding Self-contamination** – It is known that the virus (SARS-CoV-2) can also get transmitted through the objects contaminated with infectious agents (fomites). There is no way one can be sure whether the surface that he or she touched was contaminated with the pathogen or not. Touching of eyes, nose, or mouth after touching unclean surfaces with hand increases an individual's risk of getting infected. In conditions like this, it is advisable to be extra careful about the possibility of self-contamination.

4.4 CLEANING AND DISINFECTION OF SURFACES IN NONHEALTHCARE SETTINGS

The process of eliminating many or all pathogenic microorganisms (except spore-forming bacteria) from inanimate objects is known as disinfection

(CDC, 2008). The implementation of proper disinfection practices helps reduce the chances of contamination by pathogenic microorganisms (in this case, SARS-CoV-2) in nonhealthcare settings (see Figure 4.5). Nonhealthcare setting includes home, schools, colleges, offices, places for community gathering, markets, etc. Surfaces that are generally accessed by multiple people, for example, doorknobs, workstations, personal devices, windows, surfaces of bathroom and toilets, and food preparation area, known as "high-touch surfaces," should be disinfected with high priority. For disinfection purposes of nonhealthcare settings, the World Health Organization recommends the use of 0.1% sodium hypochlorite solution (bleach or chlorine). The 0.1% can be prepared by mixing 1 part of household bleach with 49 parts of normal water. For example, by mixing 1 ml of household bleach with 49 ml of water, one can make 50 ml of 0.1% sodium hypochlorite solution. Other than sodium hypochlorite, 70%–90% alcohol can also be used. The disinfectant solutions must be kept in an opaque container away from sunlight, but preparing the disinfectant solution readily before use gives better results. The World Health Organization recommends that cleaning of surfaces should begin from less dirty area to more dirty areas. Disinfection of the surfaces for COVID-19 requires the use of clothes or wipes soaked in a disinfectant solution. The World Health Organization does not recommend spraying of disinfectant for COVID-19. While using disinfectant, the following points should be kept in mind (WHO, 2020a):

- The odor from the disinfectant may cause respiratory irritation, and therefore it is advisable to keep the room well ventilated while using them.
- It is advisable to use basic PPE such as face mask, hand gloves, waterproof aprons, and closed shoes to avoid direct contact of skin with the disinfectant. The reuse of disposable items is not recommended.
- Disinfectant solutions should be kept away from the reach of the children and pets.
- Disinfectants are toxic substances and should never be used for cleaning body surfaces. It causes irritation or damage to eyes, skin, and respiratory system.
- Food substances should never be washed with disinfectants (see Chapter 6, Section 6.6).

Frequent hand washing and avoiding self-contamination should be followed as a primary prevention measure in places where regular cleaning or disinfection of surfaces is not possible (WHO, 2020a).

4.5 MAINTAINING PROPER SELF-ISOLATION AND QUARANTINE AND SEEKING MEDICAL CARE

Exposure to infectious agents or contagious diseases can be prevented (to an extent) by the implementation of proper self-isolation or quarantine measures. Self-isolation is the process of keeping people infected with contagious disease separate from healthy people. Quarantine is the process of restricting the movement of people exposed to a contagious disease to be sure whether they develop the disease or not. Social distancing is not the same as self-isolation and quarantine. Social distancing means the act of avoiding locations or situations where there is a risk of getting exposed to a contagious disease. Self-isolation should be implemented if individuals are experiencing symptoms such as mild fever, cough, or headache or if they have been tested positive for COVID-19, they are advised to self-isolate themselves at home until fully recovered (at least 7 days) (NHS, 2020) or if the individual suspects of being exposed to the COVID-19-infected person (at least 14 days) (NHS, 2020). During this self-isolation period, going out in public, letting unnecessary visitors in, contact with pets or animals must be avoided. It is important to perform proper monitoring of the symptoms. Self-isolation process should not be discontinued without the permission from healthcare providers. If the symptoms get worse and the individual experiences difficulty in breathing, it is advised to seek medical attention immediately (WHO, 2020a).

REFERENCES

Coronavirus Disease (COVID-19) Advice for the Public. World Health Organization. (2020a, June 4). Available at https://www.who.int/emergencies/diseases/novel-coronavirus-2019/advice-for-public. Accessed on June 26, 2020.

Frequently Asked Questions about Respiratory Hygiene and Cough Etiquette. Virginia Department of Health. (2011). https://www.google.com/url?sa=t&rct=j&q=&esrc=s&source=web&cd=&ved=2ahUKEwjAlYbwgsLqAhWBXisKHdlIAnkQFjABegQICxAD&url=https%3A%2F%2Fwww.vdh.virginia.gov-%2Fcontent%2Fuploads%2Fsites%2F3%2F2016%2F01%2FRespiratoryHygieneCoughEtiquette_FAQ.pdf&usg=AOvVaw1QxVjMxmLcZK86k65MrVOI. Accessed on June 30, 2020.

Hand Hygiene: Why, How & When? World Health Organization. (2009). Revised August 2009. https://www.google.com/url?sa=t&rct=j&q=&esrc=s&source= web&cd=&ved=2ahUKEwjj7MKImcXqAhVKWH0KHfDvDr8QFjABegQ IChAD&url=https%3A%2F%2Fwww.who.int%2Fgpsc%2F5may%2FHand_ Hygiene_Why_How_and_When_Brochure.pdf%3Fua%3D1&usg=AOvVaw1p 0dZQcyEDg3fxNiLBGOXE. Accessed on July 11, 2020.

Infection Prevention and Control of Epidemic- and Pandemic-prone Acute Respiratory Infections in Health Care. Geneva: World Health Organization. (2014). Available at https://apps.who.int/iris/bitstream/handle/10665/112656/9789241507134_ eng.pdf;jsessionid=41AA684FB64571CE8D8A453C4F2B2096?sequence=1).

Introduction, Methods, Definition of Terms. Guideline for Disinfection and Sterilization in Healthcare Facilities. Centers for Disease Control and Prevention. (2008). Available at https://www.cdc.gov/infectioncontrol/ guidelines/disinfection/introduction.html. Accessed on July 2, 2020.

Modes of Transmission of Virus Causing COVID-19: Implications for IPC Precaution Recommendations. World Health Organization. Scientific brief. First published on 29 March 2020b, updated on 9 July based on updated scientific evidence. (2020b). Available at https://www.who.int/news-room/commentaries/detail/ modes-of-transmission-of-virus-causing-covid-19-implications-for-ipc- precaution-recommendations. Accessed on July 11, 2020.

Standard Precautions: Hand Hygiene. World Health Organization. OpenWHO. (2020). Available at https://openwho.org/courses/IPC-HH-en. Accessed on June 21, 2020.

When to Self-Isolate and What to Do. NHS. (2020). Available at https://www.nhs. uk/conditions/coronavirus-covid-19/self-isolation-and-treatment/when-to-self- isolate-and-what-to-do/. Accessed on July 7, 2020.

Why is Washing Your Hands so Important during this Pandemic? Gavi: The Vaccine Alliance. (2020, April 17). Available at https://www.gavi.org/vaccineswork/ why-washing-your-hands-so-important-during-pandemic. Accessed on June 30, 2020.

Cutting-Edge Research to Combat COVID-19

5

5.1 INTRODUCTION

The pandemic of COVID-19 has caused fear and concern regarding the global health safety. Scientists and policymakers worldwide are currently working in collaboration to find out the evidence-based treatment and ways of implementing them in order to treat patients with COVID-19. Globally, institutions, pharmaceutical companies, universities, nongovernment organizations, and several groups of independent researchers are involved in the research and development of vaccines, new antiviral agents, medical devices, etc. (Naqvi et al., 2020). This section covers the research and development of potential investigational therapies in relation to COVID-19. It is to be understood that the research and development are progressing at a rapid pace and new data are becoming available every day, and thus the information presented here about the cutting-edge research may change over time. This section will focus mainly on vaccines, neutralizing monoclonal antibody (mAb) therapy, immunotherapies, and medical devices.

5.2 RESEARCH AND DEVELOPMENT OF VACCINES

Since the beginning of the COVID-19 pandemic, scientists worldwide are working tirelessly with the sole aim of developing a permanent treatment for COVID-19. Several kinds of approaches are being implemented and are put to trial for the vaccine development for COVID-19. Even if the scientific community is progressing with speed, the process of vaccine development takes time. It is the responsibility of vaccine regulatory authorities to make sure that the vaccine is safe for humans before it is approved for the therapeutic use. All vaccines go through a rigorous process to make sure that they are safe and effective. Vaccine effectivity and safety are assessed through clinical trials having multiple phases. Currently, there is no vaccine, treatment, or cure approved for COVID-19 as of June 30, 2020. Scientists hope to deliver approved and safe treatments for COVID-19 as early as possible. Following are the names of some potential vaccine candidates for COVID-19 that are currently under investigation:

1. **mRNA-1273** – National Institute of Allergy and Infectious Diseases and Moderna Inc. started phase 1 trial of mRNA-based vaccine (mRNA-1273) for the treatment of COVID-19. mRNA-1273 is Moderna's tenth vaccine against infectious disease to initiate clinical trials (Moderna, 2020a; Moderna, 2020b; NIH, 2020).
2. **ChAdOx1 nCoV-19 Vaccine** – Jenner Institute of Oxford University has started clinical trials in May 2020 for the testing of the ChAdOx1 nCoV-19 vaccine. The clinical trial is under progress as of June 2020 (University of Oxford, 2020).
3. **mRNA Vaccine BNT162** – Pfizer Inc. and BioNTech SE initiated clinical trial in May 2020. This trial is a part of the global development program and intends to increase the production capacity in 2021 (Pfizer, 2020).
4. **SARS-CoV-2 Vaccine** – Collaboration of Johnson and Johnson with Emergent BioSolutions and Catalent led to the utilization of manufacturing services of Janssen's AdVac and PER.C6 technologies that are known to provide rapid upscale production of an optimal vaccine candidate. According to their report, testing on healthy individuals should be initiated in July 2020. This initiative also has expanded collaboration with the Biomedical Advanced

Research and Development Authority (Johnson and Johnson, 2020).

5. **Saponin-Based Matrix M Adjuvant Vaccine (NVX-CoV2373)** – Novavax and Emergent BioSolutions have collaborated in the development of saponin-based matrix M adjuvant vaccine, which is proposed to function by stimulating the entry of antigen-presenting cell into the injection site and enhances the antigen presentation in local lymph nodes to boost the immune response. This initiative is funded by the United States Department of Defense (Novavax, 2020).

6. **INO 4800** – The phase 1 human clinical trial enrollment of 40 healthy volunteers is complete as of late April 2020. Interim results of safety and immunogenicity are expected in June. Inovio has received a grant from the Bill and Melinda Gates Foundation to accelerate testing and scale up a smart device (Cellectra 3PSP) for large-scale intradermal vaccine delivery (INOVIO, 2020).

7. **COVID-19 S-Trimer** – Preclinical development is underway using GSK's adjuvants (compounds that enhance vaccine efficacy) and Clover's proprietary proteins, which stimulate an immune response (GSK, 2020).

8. **CpG 1018 Adjuvant** – Dynavax is providing CpG 1018, the adjuvant contained in the United States Food and Drug Administration (US FDA)-approved HEPLISAV-B vaccine to support the development of Valneva's COVID-19 vaccine candidate (Dynavax, 2020).

9. **Polymerase Chain Reaction (PCR)-Based DNA Vaccine** – The collaboration has designed four COVID-19 vaccine candidates utilizing PCR-based DNA manufacturing systems for preclinical testing in animals (Pharmaceutical Technology, 2020).

10. **Nanoparticle SARS-CoV-2 Vaccine** – On March 23, 2020, Ufovax (Scripps Research) reported the development of vaccine prototype utilizing self-assembling protein nanoparticle (1c-SApNP) vaccine platform technology. 1c-SApNP was invented by Dr. Jiang Zhu at the Department of Integrative Structural and Computational Biology at Scripps Research (Ufovax, 2020).

11. **COVAXIN™** – Bharat Biotech in collaboration with the Indian Council of Medical Research and National Institute of Virology developed India's first indigenous vaccine for COVID-19. Drugs Controller General of India has approved this vaccine for Phase I and II human clinical trials, which are scheduled to begin from July 2020 across India (Bharat Biotech, 2020).

5.3 RESEARCH AND DEVELOPMENT OF ANTIBODY-DIRECTED THERAPIES

In 1986, the US FDA approved mAbs for the first time (Lu et al., 2020). mAbs are artificially synthesized proteins that function like human antibodies (American Cancer Society, 2019), which are implemented as passive immunotherapy for the treatment of viral infections. The therapeutic potential of mAbs has been well documented in the treatment of many diseases. mAbs targeted against SARS-CoV-2 possess the potential for therapeutic application (Marston et al., 2018). Researchers worldwide have isolated mAbs directed against SARS-CoV-2 mainly from B-cells of patients recovered from SARS-CoV-2 or isolated previously from SARS-CoV. Potential mAbs can also be obtained by immunizing humanized mice (Marovich et al., 2020). Humanized mice are model organisms possessing functional human genes, cells, tissues, or organs and are used in the medical research (Yong et al., 2018). Potential mAbs specific for SARS-CoV-2 recognize specific receptor-binding domains of the spike protein (Ju et al., 2020; Pinto et al., 2020). Neutralizing mAbs act by blocking the formation of spike protein–Angiotensin Converting Enzyme-2 (ACE-2) receptor complex. Knowledge obtained from studying other human coronaviruses like SARS-CoV and MERS-CoV has contributed significantly to understanding the molecular structure of spike proteins (Wrapp et al., 2020). Based on the studies performed on SARS-CoV and MERS-CoV, researchers reported that neutralizing antibodies can target other regions of the spike protein as well (Wang et al., 2018). mAbs are studied using specific culture assays (in vitro), which is very useful in selecting antibodies having the desired specificity. SARS-CoV-2 mAbs have the potential to be used for both the prevention and the treatment of infection (Marovich, 2020). mAbs provide an alternative course of action for the prevention of COVID-19. Passive implementation of mAbs as preexposure or postexposure prophylaxis might offer immediate protection from the infection that may last for weeks or months. Figure 5.1 represents the action of neutralizing antibodies in blocking SARS-CoV-2 infection.

This section points out some of the potential neutralizing antibodies that are currently undergoing the process of development and clinical trials for the treatment of COVID-19.

1. **Anti SARS-CoV-2 Polyclonal Hyperimmune Globulin (H-IG)** – Takeda Pharmaceutical Company Limited on March 4, 2020, announced their proceedings regarding plasma-derived therapy for

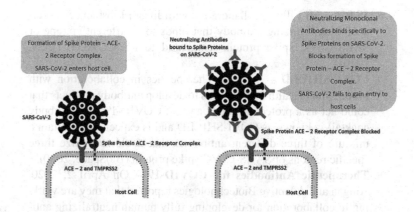

FIGURE 5.1 Blocking of SARS-CoV-2 infection by neutralizing antibodies.

COVID-19. This is currently under development, and the research-ers believe H-IG could be implemented in treating patients with high risk (Takeda, 2020).

2. **Monoclonal Antibodies** – Regeneron Pharmaceuticals, Inc. has identified several antibodies having the ability to neutralize viruses. Based on their report published on March 17, 2020, the mAb cock-tail will be implemented in human clinical trials for COVID-19. According to their report, the novel multiantibody cocktail can be administered as prophylaxis before exposure to SARS-CoV-2 or can be provided as an actual treatment to the patients suffering from COVID-19 (Regeneron, 2020).

3. **VIR-7831 and VIR-7832** – VIR Biotechnology in collaboration with Biogen and Generation Bio has developed mAbs (VIR-7831 and VIR-7832) that bind to specific epitopes present on SARS-CoV-2 (similar to epitopes of SARS-CoV). These mAbs have been engineered to have an extended half-life (Vir, 2020).

4. **Polyclonal H-IG (TAK-888)** – Takeda Pharmaceutical Company Limited is developing virus-specific antibodies (TAK-888) in con-centrated form from the plasma obtained from individuals recov-ered from COVID-19 (Takeda, 2020).

5. **LY COV555** – Eli Lilly in collaboration with AbCellera have devel-oped an investigational medicine called LY COV555, an antibody therapy for the prevention and treatment of COVID-19. According to the report published by Lilly, LY COV555 is the first potential new medicine specifically designed to attack SARS-CoV-2 (Lilly, 2020b).

6. **JS 016** – Eli Lilly in collaboration with Junshi Bioshiences developed a neutralizing antibody that binds to a different epitope of SARS-CoV-2 spike protein (compared to LY COV555) (Lilly, 2020a).

7. **COVI SHIELD** – Sorrento Therapeutics in collaboration with Mount Sinai Health System aims to develop antibody products that could act as a protective shield against COVID-19. The antibody cocktail is known as COVI-SHIELD and is expected to contain a mixture of three different antibodies that could recognize three specific regions of SARS-CoV-2 spike protein (BioSpace, 2020).

8. **Therapeutic Antibodies for COVID-19** – On April 2, 2020, Amgen and Adaptive Biotechnologies reported that they are working in collaboration for developing fully human neutralizing antibodies targeted against SARS-CoV-2 that might help prevent or treat COVID-19 (Amgen, 2020).

9. **Antibody Combination** – On June 9, 2020, AstraZeneca reported their agreement US Government Agencies regarding proceedings for developing a pair of mAbs for the prevention and treatment of COVID-19. In April 2020, Vanderbilt University (USA) has granted licensed coronavirus-neutralizing antibodies to AstraZeneca (AstraZeneca, 2020).

5.4 INVESTIGATIONAL IMMUNOTHERAPIES ASSOCIATED WITH COVID-19

The process of treating diseases by either activating or suppressing the immune system is termed as immunotherapy. Immunotherapies that enhance immune response are known as activation immunotherapy and immunotherapies that suppress immune response are known as suppression immunotherapy. This section points out some of the potential immunotherapy candidates that are currently undergoing the process of development and clinical trials for the treatment of COVID-19.

1. **LEAPS** – CEL-SCI Corporation initiated the development of immunotherapy that implements Ligand Antigen Epitope Presentation System (LEAPS) peptide technology for reducing COVID-19 viral load and associated lung damage. CEL-SCI

utilizes the LEAPS peptide approach that has the ability to elicit a cell-mediated antiviral response as well as anti-inflammatory or immunomodulatory response as documented from the studies on animals (CEL-SCI, 2020).

2. **Brilacidin** – On May 5, 2020, Innovation Pharmaceuticals reported that they enacted a material transfer agreement with Public Health Research Institute (United States) for evaluating antiviral and immunomodulatory properties of brilacidin against COVID-19. Researchers are involved in studying the inhibitory effect of brilacidin on SARS-CoV-2 replication. Samples were obtained from young and old-aged donors so that age-dependent responses can be included in the study. Several molecular screening and cellular assays revealed its antiviral property against SARS-CoV-2. Studies have shown that Brilacidin has the ability to inhibit the action of cytokines like Interleukin-1 (IL-1), Interleukin-6 (IL-6), and Tumor Necrosis Factor- α (TNF-α) and other inflammatory mediators. These evidences provide a foundation for considering brilacidin as a potential investigational therapeutic candidate in relation to COVID-19 (Innovation Pharmaceuticals Inc. 2020).

3. **Autologous, Adipose-Derived Mesenchymal Stem Cells (HB-adMSCs)** – On April 20, 2020, Hope Biosciences reported about the approval regarding the third phase of the clinical trial for COVID-19. Hope Biosciences in collaboration with Advanced Diagnostics Healthcare of River Oaks Hospital and Clinics aims in implementing HB-adMSCs safely and efficiently to COVID-19 patients. Based on the evidence obtained from ongoing studies, researchers believe that the immunomodulatory and regenerative properties of mesenchymal stem cells may help in lowering the severity of respiratory complications of COVID-19 infection (Hope Biosciences, 2020)

4. **Allogeneic Natural Killer (NK) Cells (CYNK-001)** – On April 2, 2020, Celularity Inc. reported that the US FDA has permitted the implementation of proprietary CYNK-001 on patients suffering from COVID-19. CYNK-001 is an allogeneic, NK cell therapy obtained from placental hematopoietic stem cells. The organization believes that CYNK-001 is the first investigational new drug (IND) that received clearance from the US FDA for the treatment of COVID-19. Based on the outcomes of ongoing research, CYNK-001 may provide protection form COVID-19 by disrupting the SARS-CoV-2 replication process and eliminating the infected cells (Celularity, 2020).

5. **Immune Globulin IV (Octagram 10%)** – On May 20, 2020, Octapharma USA has reported that the US FDA has approved the third-phase clinical trial for their investigational new drug (octagram 10%) for COVID-19. Octagram 10% also known as human immune globulin intravenous is human immunoglobulin used for the treatment of chronic immune thrombocytopenic purpura (Octapharma, 2020).

5.5 INVESTIGATIONAL DEVICES ASSOCIATED WITH COVID-19

1. **Blood Purification Device** – Several extracorporeal blood purification filters (e.g., CytoSorb, oXiris, Seraph 100 Microbind, Spectra Optia Apheresis) have received emergency use authorization from the FDA for the treatment of severe COVID-19 pneumonia in patients with respiratory failure. The devices have various purposes, including use in continuous renal replacement therapy or in reduction of proinflammatory cytokine levels (FDA, 2020).
2. **Nanosponges** – Engineers and researchers at the University of California San Diego and Boston University together developed

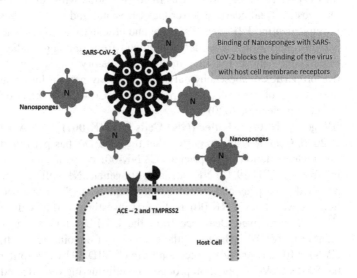

FIGURE 5.2   Nanosponges in treating COVID-19.

"nanosponges" for fighting COVID-19. The first data regarding these nanosponges is published on June 17, 2020 in *Nano Letters* (ScienceDaily, 2020). Cellular nanosponges made from plasma membranes derived from human type II lung epithelial cells or human macrophages have been studied in vitro. The nanosponges display the same protein receptors required by SARS-CoV-2 for cellular entry and binds efficiently to the virus. The binding of nanosponges with the spike protein of SARS-CoV-2 blocks the formation of spike protein–ACE-2 receptor complex. Thus the host cell stays protected (Zhang et al., 2020). Figure 5.2 represents the role of nanosponges in blocking SARS-CoV-2 infection.

REFERENCES

CEL-SCI Initiates Development of Immunotherapy to Treat COVID-19 Coronavirus Infection. (2020, March 9). Available at https://www.irdirect.net/prviewer/release_only/id/4254600. Accessed on June 26, 2020.

Celularity Announces FDA Clearance of IND Application for CYNK-001 in Coronavirus, First in Cellular Therapy. CYNK-001, the Company's Allogeneic, Off-the-Shelf, Cryopreserved Natural Killer Cell Therapy to Be Used in Phase I/II Study. CISION PR Newswire. (2020, April 2). Available at https://www.prnewswire.com/news-releases/celularity-announces-fda-clearance-of-ind-application-for-cynk-001-in-coronavirus-first-in-cellular-therapy-301034141.html. Accessed on June 26, 2020.

Clover and GSK Announce Research Collaboration to Evaluate Coronavirus (COVID-19) Vaccine Candidate with Pandemic Adjuvant System. GSK. (2020, February 24). Available at https://www.gsk.com/en-gb/media/press-releases/clover-and-gsk-announce-research-collaboration-to-evaluate-coronavirus-covid-19-vaccine-candidate-with-pandemic-adjuvant-system/#. Accessed on June 26, 2020.

COVAXINTM – India's First Indigenous COVID-19 Vaccine. Bharat Biotech. (n.d.) Available at https://www.bharatbiotech.com/covaxin.html. Accessed on July 1, 2020.

COVID – 19 Oxford Vaccine Trial. University of Oxford. (n.d.) Available at https://covid19vaccinetrial.co.uk/. Accessed on June 26, 2020.

FDA Approves Octapharma USA Investigational New Drug Application for Severe COVID-19 Patients. OctaPharma News. (2020, May 20). Available at https://www.octapharmausa.com/en/news-contact/news-single-view.html?tx_ttnews%5Btt_news%5D=1148&cHash=272a8924d90e94efcabf0d2fe596271d. Accessed on June 30, 2020.

FDA Combating COVID-19 with Medical Devices. U.S. Food and Drug Administration. (2020, June 15). Available at https://www.fda.gov/media/136702/download. Accessed on June 26, 2020.

Hope Biosciences Announces Third FDA-Approved Clinical Trial for COVID-19. Mesenchymal Stem Cells for Treatment of Hospitalized COVID-19 Patients. Hope Biosciences. (2020, April 20). Available at https://www.hope.bio/post/hope-biosciences-announces-third-fda-approved-clinical-trial-for-covid-19. Accessed on June 26, 2020.

Inhibitory Effect of Innovation Pharmaceuticals' Brilacidin on SARS-CoV-2 (COVID-19) in Primary Human Immune Cells to Be Studied at Leading Public Health Research Institute. Innovation Pharmaceuticals Inc. (2020, May 5). Available at http://www.ipharminc.com/press-release/2020/5/5/inhibitory-effect-of-innovation-pharmaceuticals-brilacidin-on-sars-cov-2-covid-19-in-primary-human-immune-cells-to-be-studied-at-leading-public-health-research-institute. Accessed on June 26, 2020.

Innovation Pharmaceuticals Brilacidin Received by U.S. Regional Biocontainment Laboratory; Testing against Coronavirus (COVID-19). Innovation Pharmaceuticals Inc. (2020, March 9). Available at http://www.ipharminc.com/press-release/2020/3/9/innovation-pharmaceuticals-brilacidin-received-by-us-regional-biocontainment-laboratory-testing-against-coronavirus-covid-19. Accessed on June 26, 2020.

INOVIO Completes Enrollment in the Phase 1 U.S. Trial of INO-4800 for COVID-19 DNA Vaccine; Interim Results Expected in June. INOVIO News Details, (2020, April 28). Available at http://ir.inovio.com/news-releases/news-releases-details/2020/INOVIO-Completes-Enrollment-in-the-Phase-1-US-Trial-of-INO-4800-for-COVID-19-DNA-Vaccine-Interim-Results-Expected-in-June/default.aspx. Accessed on June 26, 2020.

Johnson & Johnson Announces Collaboration with U.S. Department of Health & Human Services to Accelerate Development of a Potential Novel Coronavirus Vaccine. Johnson and Johnson. (2020, February 11). Available at https://www.jnj.com/johnson-johnson-announces-collaboration-with-u-s-department-of-health-human-services-to-accelerate-development-of-a-potential-novel-coronavirus-vaccine. Accessed on June 26, 2020.

Ju, B., Zhang, Q., Ge, X., et al. (2020, March 26) "Potent human neutralizing antibodies elicited by SARS-CoV-2 infection." *bioRxiv.* doi:10.1101/2020.03.21.990770.

Lilly Announces Start of a Phase 1 Study for its Second Potential COVID-19 Antibody Treatment. Lilly. (2020a, June 8). Available at https://investor.lilly.com/news-releases/news-release-details/lilly-announces-start-phase-1-study-its-second-potential-covid. Accessed on June 26, 2020.

Lilly Begins World's First Study of a Potential COVID-19 Antibody Treatment in Humans. Lilly. (2020b, June 1). Available at https://investor.lilly.com/news-releases/news-release-details/lilly-begins-worlds-first-study-potential-covid-19-antibody. Accessed on June 26, 2020.

Lu, R., Hwang, Y., Liu, I., et al. (2020). "Development of therapeutic antibodies for the treatment of diseases." *Journal of Biomedical Science*, 27 (1). DOI: 10.1186/s12929-019-0592-z.

Marovich, M., Mascola, J.R., and Cohen, M.S. (2020, June 15). "Monoclonal antibodies for prevention and treatment of COVID-19." *The Journal of the American Medical Association*, Published online. DOI:10.1001/jama.2020.10245.

Marston, H D., Paules, C.I., and Fauci, A.S. (2018). "Monoclonal antibodies for emerging infectious diseases—borrowing from history." *The New England Journal of Medicine*, 378 (16): 1469–1472.

Moderna Announces First Participant Dosed in NIH-led Phase 1 Study of mRNA Vaccine (mRNA-1273) against Novel Coronavirus. Moderna Press Releases. (2020a, March 16). Available at https://investors.modernatx.com/news-releases/news-release-details/moderna-announces-first-participant-dosed-nih-led-phase-1-study. Accessed on June 26, 2020.

Moderna and Lonza Announce Worldwide Strategic Collaboration to Manufacture Moderna's Vaccine (mRNA-1273) against Novel Coronavirus. Moderna Press Releases. (2020b, May 1). Available at https://investors.modernatx.com/news-releases/news-release-details/moderna-and-lonza-announce-worldwide-strategic-collaboration. Accessed on June 26, 2020.

Monoclonal Antibodies and Their Side Effects. Immunotherapy. American Cancer Society. (2019). Available at https://www.cancer.org/treatment/treatments-and-side-effects/treatment-types/immunotherapy/monoclonal-antibodies.html. Accessed on June 30, 2020.

Nanosponges Could Intercept Coronavirus Infection. ScienceDaily, Science News, University of California, San Diego. (2020, June 17). Available at https://www.sciencedaily.com/releases/2020/06/200617090950.htm. Accessed on June 30, 2020.

Naqvi, A. A., Fatima, K., Mohammad, T., et al. (2020). "Insights into SARS-CoV-2 genome, structure, evolution, pathogenesis and therapies: structural genomics approach." *Biochimica Et Biophysica Acta (BBA) - Molecular Basis of Disease*, 1866 (10): 165878. doi:10.1016/j.bbadis.2020.165878.

NIH Clinical Trial of Investigational Vaccine for COVID-19 Begins. Study Enrolling Seattle-Based Healthy Adult Volunteers. NIH. (2020, March 16). Available at https://www.nih.gov/news-events/news-releases/nih-clinical-trial-investigational-vaccine-covid-19-begins. Accessed on June 26, 2020.

Novavax Awarded Department of Defense Contract for COVID-19 Vaccine. Novavax Press Release. (2020, June 4). Available at http://ir.novavax.com/news-releases/news-release-details/novavax-awarded-department-defense-contract-covid-19-vaccine. Accessed on June 26, 2020.

Pfizer and BioNTech Dose First Participants in the U.S. as Part of Global COVID-19 mRNA Vaccine Development Program. Pfizer. (2020, May 5). Available on https://www.pfizer.com/news/press-release/press-releasedetail/pfizer_and_biontech_dose_first_participants_in_the_u_s_as_part_of_global_covid_19_mrna_vaccine_development_program. Accessed on June 22, 2020.

Pharmaceutical Technology, Applied DNA, Takis Biotech Design Four Covid-19 Vaccine Candidates. Applied DNA Sciences, Pharmaceutical Technology News. (2020, March 3). Available at https://www.pharmaceutical-technology.com/news/applied-dna-takis-covid-19-vaccine/. Accessed on June 26, 2020.

Pinto, D., Park, Y. J., Beltramello, M., et al. (2020, May 18). Cross-neutralization of SARS-CoV-2 by a human monoclonal SARS-CoV antibody. *Nature*. DOI: 10.1038/s41586-020-2349-y.

Rajeev Venkayya, President, Global Vaccine Business Unit on the latest on the Coronavirus and Takeda. Takeda. (2020, March 6). Available at https://www.takeda.com/newsroom/featured-topics/rajeev-venkayya-president-global-vaccine-business-unit-on-the-latest-on-the-coronavirus-and-takeda/. Accessed on June 26, 2020.

Regeneron Announces Important Advances in Novel COVID-19 Antibody Program. Regeneron. (2020, March 17). Available at https://investor.regeneron.com/news-releases/news-release-details/regeneron-announces-important-advances-novel-covid-19-antibody. Accessed on June 22, 2020.

Sorrento and Mount Sinai Team Up for Antibody Cocktail COVI-SHIELD Project. BioSpace. (2020, May 8). Available at https://www.biospace.com/article/sorrento-and-mount-sinai-team-to-develop-antibody-therapy-against-covid-19/?keywords=covi-shield. Accessed on June 26, 2020.

Takeda Initiates Development of a Plasma-Derived Therapy for COVID-19. Takeda. (2020, March 4). Available at https://emedicine.medscape.com/article/2500114-treatment#d18. Accessed on June 22, 2020.

Ufovax Successfully Extended its Nanoparticle Vaccine Technology to SARS-CoV-2. Ufovax. (2020, March 23). Available at https://www.ufovax.com/ufovax-successfully-extended-its-nanoparticle-vaccine-technology-to-sars-cov-2/. Accessed on June 26, 2020.

Valneva and Dynavax Announce Collaboration to Advance Vaccine Development for COVID-19. Dynavax. (2020, April 22). Available at http://investors.dynavax.com/news-releases/news-release-details/valneva-and-dynavax-announce-collaboration-advance-vaccine. Accessed on June 26, 2020.

Vir Biotechnology and Biogen Execute Agreement to Manufacture SARS-CoV-2 Antibodies for Potential COVID-19 Treatment. VIR Press Release Details. (2020, May 29). Available at https://investors.vir.bio/news-releases/news-release-details/vir-biotechnology-and-biogen-execute-agreement-manufacture-sars. Accessed on June 26, 2020.

Wrapp, D., Wang. N., Corbett, K. S., et al. (2020). "Cryo-EM structure of the 2019-nCoV spike in the prefusion conformation." *Science*, 367 (6483): 1260–1263.

Yong, K., Her, Z., and Chen, Q. (2018). "Humanized mice as unique tools for human-specific studies." *Archivum immunologiae et therapiae experimentalis*, 66 (4): 245–266. DOI: 10.1007/s00005-018-0506-x.

Zhang, Q., Honko, A., Zhou, J., Gong, H., Downs, S.N., Vasquez, J.H., Fang, R.H., Gao, W., Griffiths, A., and Zhang, L. (2020). "Cellular nanosponges inhibit SARS-CoV-2 infectivity." *Nano Letters*, acs.nanolett.0c02278. Advance online publication. DOI: 10.1021/acs.nanolett.0c02278.

Public Health Concerns and Issues Regarding COVID-19

6

6.1 INTRODUCTION

The spread of COVID-19 worldwide and the disorientation caused by it have made a serious impact not only on the economy but also on the physical and psychosocial wellbeing of people belonging to different age groups and socioeconomic status. Scientific communities are working tirelessly with the sole aim of developing safe vaccines and medications that can prevent or treat COVID-19. In the meantime, the healthcare sector worldwide is committed to develop specialized infrastructure and provide medical care to moderate to seriously affected COVID-19 patients in order to minimize the casualties caused by the ongoing pandemic. This commitment has significantly impacted services to other public health-related issues. This chapter points out some of the basic concerns and issues relating to public health. The following sections discuss how issues such as reproductive, maternal and child health, family planning, pregnancy and childbirth, breastfeeding, age-group-related health factors, mental health, and nutritional needs are impacted by COVID-19.

6.2 REPRODUCTIVE, MATERNAL, AND CHILD HEALTH DURING PANDEMIC (COVID-19)

6.2.1 Self-care of Sexual and Reproductive Health during Pandemic (COVID-19)

The World Health Organization defines self-care as the ability to promote and maintain health, prevent disease, and address illness or disability at the individual, familial, or community level without any help from healthcare providers (WHO, 2019; WHO, n.d.). This means anyone can practice self-care per need. The World Health Organization, in 2019, has suggested specific self-care guidelines regarding issues relating to sexual and reproductive health that includes pregnancy, caring for newborn, contraception, abortion, sexually transmitted diseases, and sexual health (WHO, 2019). This pandemic has caused a disturbance in the normal functioning of social and healthcare systems, and proper self-care practices can minimize the problems, especially in situations where complete lockdown or social distancing measures are implemented. By implementing self-care interventions, individuals can address and manage their own health issues. Self-care interventions such as good hand and respiratory hygiene do not require a direct meeting with healthcare providers. However, prescription of medications relating to hormonal contraception, abortion, or counseling during pregnancy requires direct guidance from healthcare professionals. There are various modes using which the necessary healthcare support is being provided and accessed during the pandemic (see Figure 6.1). Authentic regulatory organizations with expertise in public health provide genuine medical information, consultation, and follow-up to the common people through digital media, telephonic helplines, and online content. People can also get access to over-the-counter medical devices, medicines, basic diagnostic services, menstrual hygiene products, emergency contraceptive pills, and condoms from local pharmacies or drug stores (WHO, 2019; WHO, n.d.).

6.2.2 Contraception, Family Planning during Pandemic (COVID-19)

According to the World Health Organization, medically approved contraception methods are safe for use. Proper guidance from a medical professional

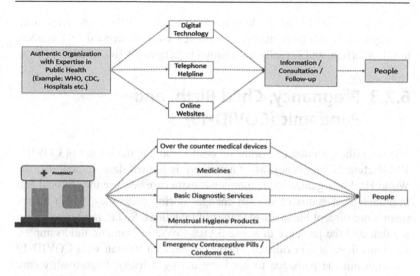

FIGURE 6.1 Modes of accessing basic healthcare information and support during pandemic.

is recommended for individuals having underlying health conditions such as diabetes, hypertension, and cancer or have delivered a baby within 6 months, etc. (consultation to be performed over the phone or digital media). To avoid pregnancy, contraceptive methods of choice that do not have medical restrictions and are easily available at the local pharmacy should be used (e.g., emergency contraceptive pills, spermicides, and condoms). Condoms help efficiently prevent unwanted pregnancy and provide protection from sexually transmitted diseases when used in a proper manner, whereas emergency contraceptive pills if taken within 5 days after intercourse can prevent pregnancy only up to 95%. In situations where the long-acting contraceptive methods (Intrauterine Contraceptive Devices [IUCDs]) need replacement after a certain period, consultation from a medical professional is recommended. Delay in the removal of long-acting methods does not cause medical complications. If due to pandemic-related restrictions, removal of long-acting devices is not feasible; it is advised that one should not try to remove the device by themselves. These processes should only be performed by an authorized healthcare provider under prescribed healthcare settings. Information and services relating to family planning are important because the sexual activity does not stop during the pandemic, and it is therefore essential that communities are provided with authentic information about the choices and possibilities that are available using which couples can make informed decisions. Contraceptive methods not only protect girls and women from negative health consequences caused by unwanted pregnancies but also help reduce additional pressure on health systems, which are working hard to address COVID-19 by preventing the negative health consequences associated with unintended pregnancies, unsafe abortion, and sexually transmitted infections (WHO, 2020c).

6.2.3 Pregnancy, Child Birth, and Pandemic (COVID-19)

The scientific community worldwide is still studying the impact of COVID-19 infection on pregnancy, as of now there is limited data. In contrast, the World Health Organization recommends extra care because the physical and immunological status of women changes during pregnancy, which makes them more susceptible to a wide range of infections. So far, researchers have not detected the presence of active SARS-CoV-2 in amniotic fluid samples. For now, there is no evidence whether a pregnant woman with COVID-19 can transmit the pathogen to her baby during delivery. High-quality care before, during, and after childbirth is the fundamental right of all pregnant women. According to the World Health Organization, the mode of birth must be chosen on the basis of the preference of the pregnant woman as well as on obstetric indications. Cesarian section is advised under medically justifiable situations. The mother can touch her newborn baby only after following proper respiratory and hand hygiene (WHO, 2016, 2018, 2020i).

6.2.4 Breastfeeding and COVID-19

According to the World Health Organization, there are no studies that report the transmission of active COVID-19 through breastfeeding. In fact, studies have shown that under all socio-economic settings, breastfeeding not only improves the health of infants but also improves maternal health (WHO, 2020b). In cases where after delivery, even if the mother is confirmed or suspected to have COVID-19, it is advised to continue skin-to-skin care as well as breastfeeding. According to the World Health Organization, skin-to-skin care improves temperature control in newborns, and breastfeeding promotes healthy development and reduces mortality. Women with confirmed or suspected COVID-19 should wear a medical mask and wash hands with soap and water before touching the baby. Even if the medical mask is not available, the World Health Organization recommends that breastfeeding should be continued because mother's milk is unquestionably essential for the physical and brain development of the baby. In situations where the mother is not able to breastfeed her baby because of complications relating to COVID-19 or any other diseases, alternative ways such as expressing milk (squeezing milk out of biological mother's breast that can be fed to the baby as per need) or donor human milk (milk donated by nursing mothers who are not biologically related) must be provided by maintaining the safety measures. If expressing breast milk or donor human milk is not available, wet nursing (another woman breastfeeds the baby) must be considered. The World Health Organization recommends not to feed infant formula milk to newborns and infants under any settings because there are always risks associated with it (WHO, 2020b).

6.3 AGE GROUP-RELATED ISSUES DURING COVID-19

6.3.1 Children

Childhood is considered the most critical period in a person's life because during this stage the physical and psychological development takes place. This makes children most vulnerable among the age groups. Physical distancing, quarantines, and complete lockdown measures implemented in response to the spread of COVID-19 have affected the physical and mental health of children worldwide. During the crisis, children may suffer from feelings of stress, anxiety, fear, and worry (WHO, 2020e). These feelings are enhanced when children are not able to interact freely as they are not able to go out and play or go to the school where they could meet their friends. Children are not used to face this kind of crisis caused due to pandemic and require extra attention and care from parents. It is to be understood that every child responds to the stress in his or her own way, and the major issue is that they often fail to express their thoughts properly (UNICEF, 2020; CDC, 2019; Child Mind Institute, 2020). It is the responsibility of the parents and caregivers to understand the behavior of their child and to ensure an environment where children can grow and develop their full potential while having fun and being healthy and safe. Parents and caregivers are advised to implement the following simple approaches (UNICEF, 2020; CDC, 2019; Child Mind Institute, 2020; WHO, 2020e):

- **Listening to Your Child** – Time is the best gift a parent or a caregiver can give to their children. Children do not know how to express their thoughts or emotions properly as adults do. They may present their issues from the level of their intellect and perspective.

It is very important that parents and caregivers must provide their children with opportunities to talk about what they are feeling. They must be encouraged to share concerns and ask questions (UNICEF, 2020; CDC, 2019; Child Mind Institute, 2020; WHO, 2020e).

- **Comforting Your Child** – Providing a comforting environment is essential. Parents and caregivers may perform activities such as storytelling, playing, or other fun and creative activities that bring mental comfort. Children should be praised frequently for their strength, such as showing courage, compassion, and helpfulness, and this helps them develop self-belief that brings a feeling of comfort in their mind (UNICEF, 2020; CDC, 2019; Child Mind Institute, 2020; WHO, 2020e).

- **Reassuring Your Child** – Children are highly dependent on their parents or caregivers. The way parents and caregivers make their children feel about them is very important. Parents and caregivers need to ensure that their children feel safe and protected under their guidance and care. Children may feel unsettled by the changes in routine or pick up on the fact that people around them are worried and upset. Children should be given the time to process any worries they may be having. The parents or caregivers should tell their child about the contribution of health workers, scientists, police, and independent groups of people worldwide who are working to stop the outbreak and keeping the community safe. Knowing that compassionate people are taking action in times of emergency brings comfort to the mind of a child (UNICEF, 2020; CDC, 2019; Child Mind Institute, 2020; WHO, 2020e).

- **Teaching Hygiene Measures** – It is important to teach your child hygiene measures in a fun and playful manner. Children must be encouraged to perform safe and hygienic practices by presenting it to them in ways they can relate to and not giving in to fear or anxiety. For example, children love to follow and copy the behavior of their favorite cartoon characters or superheroes. So presenting the lesson in the relatable and enjoyable form makes it more acceptable to them. The parents may tell their children that "Mr. Bean washes his hands properly before eating or touching his mouth, eyes, and nose." and they should follow Mr. Bean and wash their hands as well. Or "the superpower of their favorite superhero is wearing a mask and saving people from diseases" and telling your child that if they maintain good respiratory hygiene, they too will be like their favorite superhero (UNICEF, 2020; CDC, 2019; Child Mind Institute, 2020; WHO, 2020e).

- **Implementation of Creative and Positive Activities** – Introducing children to fun and creative activities such as painting, singing, and dancing not only keep them positively occupied but also help them develop skills and gain self-confidence. Positive messaging helps the children understand playfully how to stay safe during COVID-19 pandemic (UNICEF, 2020; CDC, 2019; Child Mind Institute, 2020; WHO, 2020e).
- **Protection from Unnecessary Information** – The parents and caregivers must remember that children don't need to know every little detail. Unless children ask specifically, there is no reason to provide such information that might worry them. Engaging in solution-focused thinking should be encouraged. Children should be informed (in ways suitable) about the ways fake news and wrong information can cause harm and unnecessary panic and anxiety, especially in a pandemic situation (UNICEF, 2020; CDC, 2019; Child Mind Institute, 2020; WHO, 2020e).

Children with limitations or disabilities (physical, emotional, intellectual, etc.) may have stronger reactions to the ongoing pandemic. They might suffer from more intense distress, worry, or anger because they have less control over day-to-day activities compared to other people. They require an extra word of reassurance, easily understandable explanations about the event, and more comfort and other positive reinforcements or messages. The parents and caregivers should have a conversation with them, in order to ensure their needs are taken care of and they are able to participate in all activities (UNICEF, 2020; CDC, 2019; Child Mind Institute, 2020; WHO, 2020e).

6.3.2 Adolescents, Youth

Scientific communities worldwide are still learning how COVID-19 actually affects adolescents and youths. In a process of adapting to drastic changes occurring at all socioeconomic levels, youths may succumb to the feeling of being lost and powerless leading to anxiety and depression. It is to be understood that experiencing these kinds of feelings at the time of crisis is natural and happens to everyone. In times like this, adolescents and youths need to take control of the situation by focusing on skills and strategies that help them channelize their thoughts and emotions in a productive and positive manner (see Section 6.5). Being physically active (see Section 6.4), staying connected with family and friends, and being involved in creative activities are helpful in situations like this. Adolescents and youth undergoing treatments for asthma, tuberculosis, or HIV are advised to continue their medications and attend recommended follow-ups (WHO, 2020a).

6.3.3 Old-Aged People

According to the briefings provided by the World Health Organization (April 3, 2020) on their official website, it is stated that old-aged persons possess significant risk of developing the disease, which may get severe due to aging-related physiological changes and/or underlying health conditions (WHO, 2020j). Centers for Disease Control and Prevention (CDC) also reported on their website (June 25, 2020) that 8 of 10 COVID-19 deaths in the United States have been in persons above 65 years of age (CDC, 2020). Old-aged persons above the age of 60 years are advised to take extra precaution and care in order to protect themselves against COVID-19. Some of the safety measures that need to be followed are given below:

- **Maintenance of Proper Hand and Respiratory Hygiene** – This includes washing hands thoroughly using water and soap or alcohol-based hand sanitizer as well as covering mouth and nose with a flexed elbow while sneezing or coughing. Most importantly, covering nose and mouth with an appropriate mask while meeting other people is necessary. Touching of eyes, nose, and mouth with unclean hands must be avoided (WHO, 2020h; WHO, 2020j; CDC, 2020).
- **Maintaining Proper Physical Distancing** – It is essential to keep a distance of at least 1 m with another person. Unnecessary visits to crowded places must be avoided. Restricting visitors to the house is advisable during the pandemic. In situations where allowing certain visitors are necessary (like caregivers or persons who help with daily activities), they should be asked to monitor their symptoms and maintain hand and respiratory hygiene on a regular basis before visiting (WHO, 2020h; WHO, 2020j; CDC, 2020).
- **Cleaning of Surfaces** – It is known that viruses can be present on fomites, and touching those contaminated surfaces may expose the person to the infectious agent. Frequently accessed surfaces such as doorknobs, light switches, phones, keyboards taps, and sinks should be cleaned properly using appropriate methods. Dirty surfaces should be washed with detergent and water before disinfecting (WHO, 2020h, 2020j; CDC, 2020).
- **Staying Socially Connected** – During the pandemic, it is important to be in touch with family members, caregivers, and

community care providers through phone or video calling so that they can provide help with daily activities (e.g., supply of groceries or prescription medicines or reaching out for emergency services when required) (WHO, 2020h, 2020j; CDC, 2020).

- **Identifying Secondary Caregivers** – If the old-aged person performs the responsibility of the primary caregiver to an older spouse, a child with disability, or grandchildren, then they must identify another trusted person who can take on the role of a caregiver in case the primary caregiver becomes ill (WHO, 2020h, 2020j; CDC, 2020).
- **Avoid Unnecessary News** – Continuous viewing of news updates relating to pandemic causes unnecessary anxiety and fear. News updates should be viewed only for a limited duration (WHO, 2020h, 2020j; CDC, 2020).
- **Taking Prescription Medicines** – Old-aged persons undergoing treatments for underlying health conditions are advised to continue their medications and strictly follow the instruction advised by a healthcare professional (WHO, 2020h, 2020j; CDC, 2020).

6.4 MAINTAINING PHYSICAL HEALTH DURING COVID-19

Due to the COVID-19 pandemic, people are forced to stay at home, which resulted in the reduction of physical activity. However, in a pandemic situation, it is essential that people of all age groups must perform appropriate physical activity for a particular amount of time. Simple activities like 3–4 minutes of physical movement improve blood circulation and muscle activity. Performing physical activity regularly brings body and mind at ease, which helps in reducing the susceptibility to COVID-19 by regulating underlying health conditions. Old-aged persons must perform exercises that improve their body balance. Simple breathing exercises improve physical and mental health by enriching the body with a proper amount of oxygen, activating blood circulation, and reducing the risk of depression. Physical activity if performed properly provides or improves the feeling of wellbeing (WHO, 2020g). The World Health Organization has recommended certain guidelines regarding the type and amount of physical activity required by individuals of different age groups (WHO, 2020g). Table 6.1 provides a brief idea about the requirement of physical activity per age groups.

TABLE 6.1   Requirement of physical activity of different age groups (WHO, 2020d)

AGE GROUP	RECOMMENDATIONS REGARDING PHYSICAL ACTIVITY
Infants	• To be kept physically active throughout the day. • The infants who still not have learned to move are advised to be kept on his or her stomach (tummy time) only while awake for around 30 minutes. • To be performed strictly under the supervision of parents or caregivers. • It helps baby develop strong neck and shoulder muscles and also promotes motor skills (WHO, 2020d).
Children (under 5 years)	• All young children are advised to perform at least 180 minutes of physical activity per day. • Children of 3–4 years of age are advised to reserve 60 minutes (from 180 minutes time) for physical activity of moderate to vigorous intensity (WHO, 2020d).
Children and adolescents (5–17 years)	• All children and adolescents are advised to perform at least 60 minutes of moderate- to vigorous-intensity exercises per day. • Exercises that strengthen muscles and bones to be performed 3 days per week (WHO, 2020d).
Adults (18 years and above)	• All adults are advised to perform at least 150 minutes of moderate-intensity physical activity throughout the week. • Alternatively at least 75 minutes of vigorous-intensity physical activity throughout the week. • Exercises that develop musculoskeletal strength should be performed two or more days per week (WHO, 2020d).
Old aged adults (60 years and above)	• Old-aged person having poor mobility are advised to perform exercises that help strengthen balance and prevent falls three or more days per week (depending upon their ability) (WHO, 2020d).

6.5 MAINTAINING MENTAL HEALTH DURING COVID-19

The implementation of complete lockdown and quarantine measures due to the COVID-19 pandemic has resulted in the pressing need of introducing huge and impactful changes in our daily life. Adapting one's lifestyle according to the drastically changing situations such as working from home, facing unexpected unemployment (temporary/permanent), accessing education from home, and absence of physical contact with family and friends is a challenging task for everyone (irrespective of all age groups). Other than these issues, there is constant fear and worry regarding a completely new disease that does not even have proper treatment so far. The "uncertainty" and "unknown" are the two aspects associated with COVID-19 pandemic that is nurturing the fear, anxiety, and stress leading to a deterioration of mental health among individuals of different age groups irrespective of socioeconomic status. In this crisis, it is very important to take care of one's mental health (WHO, 2020f). There are several simple measures that one can implement to maintain sound mental health for himself or herself or for those who need extra care and support.

- **Staying Up to Date** – The information regarding COVID-19 and situation reports is changing at regular intervals. In this scenario, it is important to stay informed about the updated information because it helps in realizing the reality of the ongoing situation. The information and guidelines should be obtained from trusted sources such as the World Health Organization (www.who.int), National and Local Authorities, or other trusted agencies such as News Channels or News on Radio as well as social media updates from authorized organizations (WHO, 2020f).
- **Avoiding Unnecessary News** – Just as staying updated about the situation is important, one must make sure that it must not overburden his or her mental health. It is important to know when to stop. Listening to too much news makes an individual feel anxious and distressed, which may affect mental health. It is advised to seek news updates only at specific times a day (once or twice) (WHO, 2020f).
- **Maintaining a Routine** – By maintaining proper routine and self-discipline, an individual can stay focused and organized. This helps an individual adapt to possible changes without disturbing the overall balance between work and life (WHO, 2020f).
- **Maintaining Social Connection** – In the time when movement or physical contact is restricted, it is important to stay in touch with family, friends, and colleagues through alternative means such as social media, phone calls, and video calls. Keeping touch with loved ones and sharing thoughts calms the mind and helps reduce the anxiety and stress caused by the ongoing crisis (WHO, 2020f).

- **Taking Break from the Nonproductive Habit-Forming Activities** – Being active on social media, playing videogames, and watching online shows or movies are nonproductive habit-forming activities. In the time when people are forced to stay at home, the possibility of spending more than the required amount of time with nonproductive habit-forming activities increases (WHO, 2020f). Most importantly, at the present time, the majority of the shows or video games portray sexually explicit content, extreme violence, and spreads unethical messages that are meant to cripple the mental health of individuals belonging to different age groups. These habits, in the long run, make an individual mentally and physically inactive as well as emotionally unstable, which produces a negative impact on their personal and social life. So it is important to restrict one's indulgence toward nonproductive habit-forming activities and instead of getting involved in creative and productive activities that develop his or her self-esteem and confidence (WHO, 2020f).
- **Avoiding Substance Abuse** – Just like nonproductive habit-forming activities, during lockdown situations, the possibility of indulging oneself to substance abuse (substance use disorders [SUDs]) increases. The persistent feeling of fear, anxiety, and isolation increases an individual's compulsion to resort to addictive substances such as alcohol, tobacco, and other psychoactive drugs, which in turn increases the risk of relapse. Studies have shown that individuals with SUD are more susceptible to the outcomes associated with COVID-19 (Dubey, 2020). In such situations, it is advisable to seek proper help from a medical professional and support groups (WHO, 2020f).
- **Helping, Supporting, and Caring for Others** – Studies showed that helping others boosts mental health and overall wellness by reducing stress and increasing self-esteem. During the crisis, helping the needy people in the community is a positive gesture that brings peace to the mind and thus maintains a healthy mental state (WHO, 2020f).
- **Taking Prescription Medicines** – If an individual is undergoing treatment for the underlying mental condition (clinical depression, anxiety disorder, dementia, SUD, gaming, gambling disorder, etc.), it is advisable to continue prescription medications as directed. Periodical counseling and follow-ups with mental health professionals can be performed through digital platforms.

Telemedicine may be implemented, which refers to the practice of caring for patients remotely when the provider and patient are not physically present with each other (WHO, 2020f).

6.6 MAINTAINING PROPER NUTRITION AND FOOD SAFETY DURING COVID-19

During the pandemic (COVID-19), it is essential to consume a healthy diet. The body's ability to prevent, combat, and recover from a particular disease is directly dependent on the type and quality of food that are consumed. Foods are more than just "food", it is the component that builds the foundation of the state of health. Proper diet helps boost the body's immunity, which is the only component that protects an individual from invading pathogens. Table 6.2 provides a brief idea about the general nutritional requirement for maintaining a sound health (WHO, 2020d).

Just like proper selection and consumption of nutrient-rich food substances, maintaining proper kitchen hygiene is another equally important factor for staying healthy. The food contains various kinds of microorganisms. Some of the microorganisms are pathogenic and causes foodborne diseases (e.g., stomach pain, fever, vomiting, diarrhea, etc.). The group of pathogenic microorganisms requires food, water time, and appropriate temperature for their proliferation. By implementing basic kitchen hygiene measures, these

TABLE 6.2 General nutritional requirement for maintaining the state of health

1. Consuming different varieties of fruits and vegetables
   - Mixture of whole grains, legumes and beans, and fresh fruits and vegetables to be consumed everyday adequately and liberally.
   - It is advised to consume unprocessed whole grains, legumes, fruits, and vegetables (WHO, 2020d).
2. Reduction of salt consumption
   - The amount of salt intake to be reduced to ~5 g or one tablespoon per day.
   - Canned or dried foods contain excessive amount of salt and preservatives and therefore its consumption should be reduced.
   - Food having low sodium content should be included (WHO, 2020d).

(Continued)

TABLE 6.2 (*Continued*)   General nutritional requirement for maintaining the state of health

3. Fats and oils should be taken in moderation
   - Lard, butter, and ghee should be replaced with healthier alternatives (e.g., olive oil, sunflower oil, corn oil, etc.)
   - White meat (poultry and fish) with low amount of fats should be consumed.
   - Consumption of red meat or any kind of processed meat must be avoided.
   - Low fat milk or dairy products should be consumed.
   - Processed, baked, and fried foods and foods having industrially synthesized trans fats must be avoided (WHO, 2020d).
4. Reducing the intake of sugar
   - Consumption of sweet, sugary, and fizzy drinks must be avoided.
   - Cookies, cakes, and chocolates should be replaced with fresh sweet fruits.
   - Desserts containing low amount of sugar (prepared at home) can be consumed.
   - Parents should not allow their children (especially under 2 years of age) to consume sugary food items (WHO, 2020d).
5. Consuming plenty of water
   - Water is a silent nutrient. Staying properly hydrated is essential for maintaining the optimal health.
   - Consumption of carbonated beverages or packaged sweetened drinks should be avoided strictly (WHO, 2020d).

pathogenic microorganisms can be eliminated (WHO, 2020d). The World Health Organization has recommended five simple kitchen hygiene measures called "5 Keys to Safer Food," which can be easily implemented in daily life. Table 6.3 provides a basic idea about the safety measures recommended by the World Health Organization (WHO, 2006).

Thus maintaining proper kitchen hygiene is very essential for the prevention of various kinds of food-borne illnesses. It is to be understood that nutrients present in the food do not kill SARS-CoV-2, but the consumption of nutritious food strengthens our immune system (immunonutrition), and a strong immune system is the key component that has the ability to protect an individual against invading pathogens.

Choose the Food that Nurtures and Strengthens Your Immunity and Not the Disease

TABLE 6.3 Five Keys to Safer Food as Recommended by World Health Organization (WHO, 2006)

	WORLD HEALTH ORGANIZATION (FOOD SAFETY): FIVE KEYS TO SAFER FOOD	
S. NO.	THINGS TO DO	REASON
Key-1	Keeping clean • Washing of hands is advisable before handling of food and often during the food preparation. • Washing of hands after going to toilet before resuming the food preparation. • All the surfaces and equipment to be used for the food preparation should be thoroughly washed and sanitized. • Food materials and kitchen should be kept protected from insects, pests, or other animals.	• Pathogenic microorganisms present on food causes diseases in human beings. • These pathogenic microorganisms may get transferred to the utensils, wiping cloth, and other kitchen surfaces through the hand of the person handling those food items. • The contamination increases the risk of food-borne illnesses. • Implementation of "Key-1" helps in the prevention of contamination and reduces the risk of food-borne illnesses.
Key-2	Separating raw and cooked • Poultry, raw meat, and seafood should be kept separated from other food items. • For handling raw meat or seafood, separate equipment and utensils should be used.	• Raw meat, seafood, and their juices possess higher chances of being contaminated with pathogenic microorganisms. • Keeping them along with other food materials increases the risk of cross-contamination. • Implementation of "Key-2" helps in the prevention of cross-contamination.

(Continued)

TABLE 6.3 (Continued)   Five Keys to Safer Food as Recommended by World Health Organization (WHO, 2006)

WORLD HEALTH ORGANIZATION (FOOD SAFETY): FIVE KEYS TO SAFER FOOD

S. NO.	THINGS TO DO	REASON
Key-3	Cooking thoroughly • Food items such as egg, poultry, meat, and seafood should be cooked for a longer duration. • While cooking food, the temperature should reach ~70°C. Thermometer can be used. • Cooked food should be thoroughly reheated before the consumption.	• Studies have shown that cooking food at temperature higher than 70°C destroys potential pathogenic microorganisms. • Implementation of "Key-3" makes the food safe for the consumption.
Key-4	Keeping food at safe temperature • Cooked foods should not be kept at room temperature for more than 2 hours. • All cooked and perishable food items should be refrigerated below 5°C. • Before serving, the cooked food should have temperature above 60°C.	• Microorganisms grow very quickly at room temperature. • Studies have shown that keeping food below 5°C or above 60°C lowers or stops the growth of microorganisms. • Implementation of "Key-4" helps in preventing the growth of microorganisms, thus reducing the risk of food-borne illnesses.
Key-5	Using safe water and raw materials • Clean water should be used for washing and food preparation. • Raw fruits or vegetables should be washed thoroughly before the consumption. • Fresh and wholesome foods should be selected.	• Food materials and water contaminated with pathogenic microorganisms or toxic chemicals are dangerous for human health. • Thorough washing of raw fruits and vegetables removes microorganisms or toxic chemicals. • Implementation of "Key-5" helps in the removal of toxic chemicals and pathogenic microorganisms.

REFERENCES

Adolescents, Youth and COVID-19. World Health Organization. (2020a, May 4). Available at https://www.who.int/news-room/q-a-detail/q-a-for-adolescents-and-youth-related-to-covid-19. Accessed on June 30, 2020.

Breastfeeding and COVID-19, Scientific Brief. World Health Organization. (2020b, June 23). Available at https://www.who.int/publications/i/item/10665332639. Accessed on June 30, 2020.

Caring for Children in a Disaster. Helping Children Cope with Emergencies. (2019, October 11). Centers for Disease Control and Prevention. Available at https://www.cdc.gov/childrenindisasters/helping-children-cope.html. Accessed on June 30, 2020.

Contraception/Family Planning and COVID-19. World Health Organization. (2020c, April 6). Available at https://www.who.int/emergencies/diseases/novel-coronavirus-2019/question-and-answers-hub/q-a-detail/contraception-family-planning-and-covid-19. Accessed on June 30, 2020.

Coronavirus Disease 2019 (COVID-19). Older Adults. Centers for Disease Control and Prevention. (2020, June 25). Available at https://www.cdc.gov/coronavirus/2019-ncov/need-extra-precautions/older-adults.html. Accessed on June 30, 2020.

Five Keys to Safer Food Manual. World Health Organization. (2006). Available at https://www.who.int/foodsafety/publications/5keysmanual/en/. Accessed on June 30, 2020.

HealthyAtHome – Healthy Diet. Connecting the World to Combat Coronavirus. World Health Organization. (2020d). Available at https://www.who.int/campaigns/connecting-the-world-to-combat-coronavirus/healthyathome/healthyathome---healthy-diet. Accessed on June 30, 2020.

HealthyAtHome - Healthy Parenting. World Health Organization. Advice for Public. (2020e). Available at https://www.who.int/campaigns/connecting-the-world-to-combat-coronavirus/healthyathome/healthyathome---healthy-parenting. Accessed on July 10, 2020.

HealthyAtHome – Mental Health. Connecting the World to Combat Coronavirus. World Health Organization. (2020f). Available at https://www.who.int/campaigns/connecting-the-world-to-combat-coronavirus/healthyathome/healthyathome---mental-health. Accessed on June 30, 2020.

HealthyAtHome - Physical Activity. Connecting the World to Combat Coronavirus. World Health Organization. (2020g). Available at https://www.who.int/news-room/campaigns/connecting-the-world-to-combat-coronavirus/healthyathome/healthyathome---physical-activity. Accessed on June 30, 2020.

Older People and COVID-19. World Health Organization. (2020h, May 8). Available at https://www.who.int/news-room/q-a-detail/q-a-on-on-covid-19-for-older-people. Accessed on June 30, 2020.

Pregnancy, Childbirth and COVID-19. World Health Organization. (2020i, March 18). Available at https://www.who.int/emergencies/diseases/novel-coronavirus-2019/question-and-answers-hub/q-a-detail/q-a-on-covid-19-pregnancy-and-childbirth. Accessed on June 30, 2020.

Psychosocial Support for Children during COVID – 19. A Manual for Parents and Caregivers. CHILDLINE, UNICEF India. (2020). Available at https://www.unicef.org/india/reports/psychosocial-support-children-during-covid-19. Accessed on June 30, 2020.

Sexual and Reproductive Health. What do We Mean by Self-Care? World Health Organization. (n.d.). Available at https://www.who.int/reproductivehealth/self-care-interventions/definitions/en/. Accessed on June 30, 2020.

Supporting Kids during the Coronavirus Crisis. Tips for Nurturing and Protecting Children at Home. Rae Jacobson. Child Mind Institute. (2020). Available at https://childmind.org/article/supporting-kids-during-the-covid-19-crisis/. Accessed on July 8, 2020.

WHO Consolidated Guideline on Self-Care Interventions for Health: Sexual and Reproductive Health and Rights. World Health Organization. (2019). Available at https://www.who.int/reproductivehealth/publications/self-care-interventions/en/. Accessed on June 20, 2020.

WHO Delivers Advice and Support for Older People during COVID-19. World Health Organization. Scientific Briefing. (2020j, April 3). Available at https://www.who.int/news-room/feature-stories/detail/who-delivers-advice-and-support-for-older-people-during-covid-19. Accessed on June 30, 2020.

WHO Recommendations on Antenatal Care for a Positive Pregnancy Experience. World Health Organization. (2016). Available at https://www.who.int/reproductivehealth/publications/maternal_perinatal_health/anc-positive-pregnancy-experience/en/. Accessed on June 20, 2020.

WHO Recommendations: Intrapartum Care for a Positive Childbirth Experience [Guidelines]. World Health Organization. (2018, July 9). Available at https://www.who.int/publications/i/item/9789241550215. Accessed on June 20, 2020.

WHO Recommendations: Non-clinical Interventions to Reduce Unnecessary Caesarean Sections. World Health Organization. (2018). Available at https://www.who.int/reproductivehealth/publications/non-clinical-interventions-to-reduce-cs/en/. Accessed on June 20, 2020.

COVID-19 and Environmental Perspectives

7

7.1 INTRODUCTION

COVID-19 or a novel coronavirus is a near unstoppable killer and is an emerging and rapidly evolving medical emergency situation across the globe. This gigantic viral outbreak was declared to be a Public Health Emergency of an international concern on January 30, 2020. World Health Organization (WHO) has declared the novel coronavirus disease, COVID-19 (2019-nCOV), to be a global pandemic on March 11, 2020, and until July 14, 2020 (14:00 IST), the total number of COVID-19 cases globally is 13,249,575 with 4,955,424 active cases, 575,844 deaths, and 7,718,307 recoveries. The death rate is 4.35%, and the recovery rate is 58.25%, and the figures are rapidly changing every second. In India, the total numbers of cases are 908,258 with 312,242 active cases, 23,736 deceased, and 572,280 recovered over time (all figures are recorded until 14:00 IST July, 14, 2020) and it is breaking new records everyday.

This apocalyptic global public health emergency scenario started with a reporting of pneumonia with an unknown cause in WHO country office located in Wuhan, Hubei province, in People's Republic of China (PRC) on December 31, 2019. The clinical characteristics of the infection are very similar to viral pneumonia. Respiratory sample analysis by PRC Centers for Disease Control and Prevention confirmed that the infection is related to novel coronavirus pneumonia and was caused by coronavirus (Huang et al., 2020. WHO officially named this viral outbreak as COVID-19 and International Committee on Taxonomy of Viruses ascribed it as SARS-CoV-2, the abbreviation for severe acute respiratory syndrome coronavirus-2, a member of large β-coronavirus family widely prevalent in nature. The extremely high transmissibility and infectivity despite comparatively low mortality rates make SARS-CoV-2 a unique member of the family with severe acute respiratory syndrome (SARS) and MERS (Liu et al., 2020). The crude mortality ratio (the number of reported deaths divided by the number of reported cases) is between 3% and 4%, while the infection mortality rates (the number of reported deaths by the number of infections) is comparatively lower (COVID-19 Situation Report-46, WHO). COVID-19 and influenza viruses have similar disease representation, but the speed of transmission is completely different between the two. Influenza has a shorter median incubation period (time from infection to appearance of symptoms) and a shorter serial interval of just 3 days (the time between the successive cases) in comparison with COVID-19 with a serial interval of 5–6 days. The basic reproductive number R_0 (the number of secondary infections generated from a single individual in completely susceptible populations without any interventions) is much higher in COVID-19 (2–2.5) with respect to influenza. However, Wu, Leung et al. (2020) estimated R_0 of SARS-CoV-2 to be 2.47–2.86, whereas that of SARS-CoV is 2.2–3.6 (Lipsitch et al., 2003) and MERS-CoV is 2.0–6.7 (Majumder et al., 2014). This indicates high transmissible character of 2019 n-CoV. The median age of population susceptible to SARS-CoV-2 is 47.0 years; however, the numbers are rapidly changing worldwide as new areas are being covered by the viral outbreak (Guan et al., 2020; Wu, Leung et al., 2020). Source of infection, routes of transmission, and susceptibility are three major epidemiological parameters of coronavirus family (Barreto et al., 2006) and find no exception in COVID-19. The nature and pathogenic representations between these epidemiologically linked viral diseases are contextual, and time-specific making directs comparisons an uphill task for the researchers worldwide. Genome analysis conclusively claimed that the novel coronavirus (SARS-CoV-2) has emerged from bat SARS coronavirus (SARSr-CoV-RaTG13) with complete genome recognition rates of 79.5% and 96%, respectively (Chen et al., 2020). This finding finds the basis as the detection of Group 1 coronaviruses in bats was initially observed in North America by Dominguez et al. (2007). SARS-CoV-2 isolated from pangolins and the viral strains currently infecting humans show 99% similarity per macrogenomic sequencing analysis performed by Xu et al. (2020). Emerging diseases such as COVID-19 are majorly zoonoses caused by ssRNA viruses (Woolhouse, 2002; Woolhouse and Gowtage-Sequeria, 2005). They lack proof reading activity and show spontaneous mutation and sporadically jump across the species defying all rules of evolutionary principles. The case in evidence is the COVID-19 infection of big cats (tigers and lions) of Bronx Zoo from the zookeeper who tested positive. Human to animal routes of viral transmission is not only rare but striking. Pathogenic mechanisms of SARS-CoV-2 reveal uncanny similarities with SARS-CoV. Receptor-binding domain instigates

SARS-CoV-2 to bind with angiotensin-converting enzyme 2 (ACE2) exactly in the same manner as SARS-CoV (Hoffmann et al., 2020). However, the structural model analysis conclusively confirms the binding affinity of SARS-CoV-2 is ten times more than that of SARS (Wrapp et al., 2020). Coronavirus recognizes the corresponding receptor on the target cell through the S protein on its surface and enters the cell switching on the pathogenic cytotoxicity. The high binding affinity of SARS-CoV-2 with ACE2 might help solving the crucial puzzle in using soluble ACE2 as a potential candidate for COVID-19 epidemiological treatments. In-depth annotation analysis of novel coronavirus (2019-nCoV), genome has revealed significant differences between 2019-nCoV and SARS or other members of beta-coronavirus family. Comparisons reveal 380 amino acid substitutions between these coronaviruses, which may have caused functional differences, pathogenic divergence, and increased infectivity of 2019-nCoV (Wu, Peng et al., 2020). The global viral outbreak targets elderly male patients with chronic underlying health complications such as diabetes, hypertension, coronary heart diseases, lung complications, cancers, and kidney failures more than their female counterparts (Chen et al., 2020). The commonest clinical symptoms include fever (87.9%), cough (67.7%), fatigue (38.1%), diarrhea (3.7%), and vomiting (5.0%). However, these are major symptoms and might be compounded with several other minor symptoms as developed in patients with different epidemiological fates (Guan et al., 2020; Jin et al., 2020). Acute respiratory distress syndrome (ARDS) is common among COVID-19 patients (Huang et al., 2020; Chen et al., 2020) and need not be confused with any other parallel epidemiological phenomenon. Other manifestations include abnormal neurological functions (Mao et al., 2020), renal, and hepatic anomalies (Huang et al., 2020; Wu, Song et al., 2020; Kumar, et al., 2020). Detection of the viral nucleic acid (ss-RNA) is the only noninvasive procedure of COVID-19 diagnosis, which includes the collection of swab samples from nose and throat. PRC NHCot (2020) has laid down the 2019 n-CoV pneumonia diagnosis and treatment plan. Maintenance of personal hygiene and safety, social distancing, self-isolation, quarantine of suspected individuals, and the treatment of infected ones with aggravated epidemiological risks with supplementary oxygen and mechanical ventilator support forms the basic pathway to contain COVID-19 infections globally in the absence of specific vaccine and medicine to treat COVID-19. Remdesivir, 1′-cyano-substituted adenosine nucleotide analogue, is an intravenous drug with broad-spectrum antiviral activity that inhibits viral replication through the premature termination of RNA transcription and has shown prominent in vitro activity against SARS-CoV-2 as well as other members of beta-coronavirus family per preliminary investigations conducted by US National Library of Medicine, National Institutes of Health, Health and Human Services, and a report published by Amirian et al. (2020).

Some potential success results regarding critical patient treatments have also been achieved with the usage of drugs such as hydroxychloroquine and azithromycin in Jaipur, India, but conflicting research reports are published by French researchers (Gautret et al., 2020a, 2020b; Molina et al., 2020).

The scientific investigations connecting the dots between environmental and epidemiological links of COVID-19 infections are still in its infancy and require systematic, holistic, and global research networking during the post-COVID-19 emergency. Environmental dynamics including changing climate scenarios across the world and associated anthropogenic stress factors play a significant role in the pathogenicity of macroparasites such as mosquitoes, flies, ticks, and bugs. It has been mentioned in scientific investigations as well (Remais et al., 2010). The impact of changing climate and anthropogenic factors on microorganisms, however, is not well documented (Chakravorty et al., 2020). Strong correlations between COVID-19 infections in susceptible populations and anthropogenically derived environmental toxicity affecting global populations cannot be ruled out and needs immediate understanding through the global research networking in a post-COVID-19 world. This will give us impetus in fighting global pandemics more scientifically and holistically in coming times unlike the ongoing COVID-19 pandemic trauma that grips mankind.

7.1 ENVIRONMENTAL TOXICITIES MIGHT ENCOURAGE SUSCEPTIBILITY TO COVID-19 PANDEMIC: A BRIEF COMMENTARY

Environmental toxicants leave behind unimaginable environmental damage and human health hazards of unmanageable proportions. Toxicants include broad-range xenobiotics such as pesticides, radioactive elements, chemicals, drugs, and heavy metals, which are non-biodegradable and persistent in ecosystems even under extreme conditions. Heavy metal toxicity in the environment is a globally emergent issue that is ubiquitous across all ecosystems on this planet (Tchounwou, 2012). Recent years have seen ever increasing ecological and global public health concern associated with environmental contamination by heavy metals such as lead, cadmium, chromium, and mercury. These metals have known toxicological effects and epidemiological implications on human health. Lead, for example, causes known poisoning effects on almost every organ systems of human body (Flora et al., 2012; Wani et al., 2015) and has been long regarded as one of the most dangerous environmental contaminants (Mahaffey et al., 1990). Similar toxicological reports have been generated for cadmium, chromium, and mercury. Potential health risk of cadmium has been well highlighted in the scientific literature since long and researchers worldwide have expressed deep concerns against health hazards that might lead to fatal complications. Groundwater contaminated with arsenic and cadmium was revealed in China long back (Wang et al., 2011). This study further opines that although the arsenic and cadmium concentrations in groundwater sources are well below the recommended limits of Water Quality Standards for Drinking Water (GB5749-1006) in China, but the residents served by almost all centralized drinking water sources face significant health complications including cancer. Immunocompromised patients including people with respiratory ailments, HIV patients, transplant recipients, and urban patients with health complications have shown increased tendency of viral infections (Englund et al., 2011). This include respiratory syncytial virus, influenza, and parainfluenza viruses, adenoviruses, rhinoviruses, and coronaviruses have been detected worldwide in transplant recipients and people with opportunistic infections; two third of which include acquired heavy metal toxicities. Newly identified viruses such as human metapneumoviruses (HMPVs) (Peret et al., 2002; Boivin et al., 2002), new strains of coronaviruses (Milano et al., 2010), and bocaviruses have also been detected in the symptomatic transplant recipients (Schenk et al., 2007). Community-acquired respiratory viruses (CARVs) cause significant health complications leading to morbidity and mortality among immune-compromised patients across the world. Similar findings were substantiated during the recent COVID-19 outbreak. Upper Respiratory Tract Infections (URTIs) and lower respiratory tract infections are commonly reported in CARV-dominated patients; a similar observation was also reported from the victims of COVID-19 worldwide.

Environmental toxicity acquired through air pollution in populated and heavily commuted cities of the world such as New York, London, Hong Kong, Shanghai, Beijing, New Delhi, Tokyo, Kolkata, and Moscow shows opportunistic health complications in both adults and children exposing them more to the risk of emerging and rapidly evolving pandemics under the global climate change scenarios. Heavy metal such as chromium finds way to human health hazards through vehicular pollution, industrial fumes, and cigarrate smoking. Chromium is a potent carcinogen primarily through the inhalation exposure in occupational settings (Costa and Klein, 2006). Hexavalent cadmium toxicity is majorly caused by cigarrate smoking and bad air pollution causing unparalleled damage to the respiratory and cardiac systems making COVID-19 infections more susceptible. The most important toxic effects, after contact, inhalation, or ingestion of hexavalent chromium compounds include dermatitis, allergic, and eczematous skin reactions, skin and mucous membrane ulcerations, perforation of the nasal septum, allergic asthmatic reactions, bronchial carcinomas, gastroenteritis, hepatocellular deficiency, and renal oligoanuric deficiency. The underlying health issues open doors to various other secondary epidemiological conditions including increased susceptibility toward viral infections including COVID-19. It is observed that the majority of smoking populations with COVID-19 infections have to swim upstream in their life battle against the viral pathogenicity.

Mercury is a silent killer and the most toxic of all heavy metals found commonly in several industrial, agricultural, domestic, and technological applications. Increased human exposure to heavy metals such as mercury has resulted in the exponential increase of induced toxicities such as neurological disorders, reproductive ailments, male sterility, teratogenicity, lung ailments, and dermatological complications. Increased cases of child mortality and miscarriage among urban women are a result of such secondary toxicities that do not find proper clinical investigations due to lack of awareness, low or no reported forensic cases, and of course socioeconomic as well as political inequalities. Approximately, 20,000 tons/year of mercury is added by anthropogenic activity (Hansen and Dasher, 1997). It is estimated that the mercury emissions will increase at a rate of 5% a year (Zhang et al., 2002). Low-dose mercury toxicity in human health is well documented by Zahir et al. (2005). Multiple pathways of mercury operate in the ecosystem including soil, air, and water, and almost all elements of biosphere thus further complicate the problem of mercury toxicity. Mercury toxicity is well prevalent in industrial areas (Panda et al., 1992) and also in freshwater ecosystems across the world, which is our main source of potable water (Sharma and Bhattacharya, 2016). Several researches reconfirmed the presence of lead, cadmium, chromium, and mercury in vegetables, food crops, and fishes (Dutta, Amin et al., 2017; 2018; 2019; Mallik et al., 2017). Climate change-induced acidification has aggravated the detrimental effects of the heavy metals in human health and ecosystems in general (Dutta et al., 2020). Experimental findings from East Kolkata Wetlands (EKW), a prominent Ramsar Site and a wetland of international importance, conclusively prove the bioaccumulation pattern of heavy metals both in ambient media (water and soils) and in harvested crops and fishes, which form a major food basket for the people of Kolkata. Thus, we are consuming poison every day and exposing our health systems to opportunistic infections and viral outbreaks such as COVID-19. Any sustainable strategy to combat COVID-19 must ensure bioremediation of heavy metals from our ecosystems as well as a cleaner environment for all of us to live and breathe. Else, we must prepare ourselves for many such COVID-19 pandemic disasters in the upcoming days. Global phenomena of climate change, varying weather conditions, anthropogenic stress factors, an immune-compromised body, poison in our plates, and dangerously polluted air, water, and soil would only make all the biotic components on earth including humans vulnerable to such viral outbreaks. Pre- and post-COVID-19 world would be very different due to changing socioeconomic-political scenarios and post-disaster situations. The utter chaos, psychological trauma, economic recession, joblessness, food insecurity, and most importantly unthinkable poverty in meeting basic resource needs would lead to cacophony and pandemonium of humongous proportions. Environmental management and, most importantly, handling and the usage of xenobiotics in our daily life must not take a backseat and must be included in the post-COVID-19 disaster mitigation plan for every country across the world under the leadership of WHO and other competent authorities with the global presence. Sustainable management of environment would only ensure a most powerful battle against all diseases, not only viral outbreaks. With global climate change issues hovering over us, environment and human health must be the subject of our primary and pivotal concern. Natural selection accepts the most tolerant of all species, neither the strongest and nor the weakest, as Darwin's theory goes. Our only way out from the evolving and emerging crisis situation is fulfillment of the sustainable development goals. This would help us to get back in track winning over the crisis situations exposed by natural disasters, anthropogenic pollution, and other stress factors, disease outbreaks, and several other underlying health conditions on a global scale. Figure 7.1 depicts the diagrammatic representation of fate of heavy metals in ecosystems and the possible linkages with COVID-19.

7.2 IMPACT OF COVID-19-RELATED SHUTDOWN ON ATMOSPHERIC CARBON DIOXIDE LEVEL IN KOLKATA: A CASE STUDY

We have sampled carbon dioxide in selected stations of Kolkata metropolis city during the longest and strictest lockdown imposed by Government of India to break the chain of community transmission of COVID-19. Our analysis put forward some eye-opening observations. The lockdown phase exhibited a significant decrease in CO_2 level in all the selected sites. All the selected sites are the busiest and most polluted locations of the city during normal times. The decrease percentage ranged from 24.56 (at Deshbandhu Park) to 45.37 (at Sealdah station), which may be attributed to the presence of different activities and vegetation in the respective sites (Table 7.1). The prevailing air quality in all the selected sites (as documented from the data bank of Aril 2019) also has a role to evaluate the percent decrease of CO_2 in these sites.

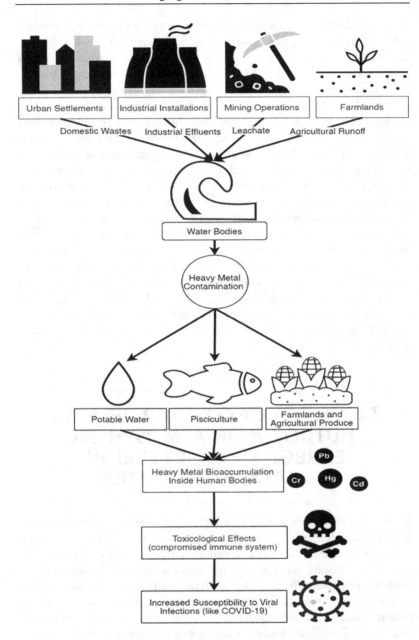

FIGURE 7.1   Diagrammatic representation of heavy metal toxicity and COVID-19 linkages in the susceptible population.

TABLE 7.1 Level of atmospheric CO_2 (in ppm) and percent decrease of CO_2 at 12 sites in the city of Kolkata during 2019 and 2020

SITES	COORDINATES	ATMOSPHERIC CO_2 (PPM)		% DECREASE OF CO_2
		2 APRIL, 2019	24 APRIL, 2020	
Laketown Crossing	22°36'02.9"N; 88°24'22.7"E	390	238	38.97
Karunamoyee Crossing	22°35'08.5"N; 88°25'18.3"E	401	247	38.40
Techno India University, WB, India	22°34'32.8"N; 88°25'43.1"E	396	230	41.92

(Continued)

TABLE 7.1 (*Continued*) Level of atmospheric CO_2 (in ppm) and percent decrease of CO_2 at 12 sites in the city of Kolkata during 2019 and 2020

| SITES | COORDINATES | ATMOSPHERIC CO_2 (PPM) | | % DECREASE OF CO_2 |
		2 APRIL, 2019	24 APRIL, 2020	
 Ballygunge Phari	22°31′32.6″N; 88°21′58.7″E	408	241	40.93
 Park Circus	22°32′21.1″N; 88°21′55.1″E	402	237	41.04
 Nabanna	22°33′55.4″N; 88°18′55.2″E	399	226	43.36

(Continued)

TABLE 7.1 (*Continued*) Level of atmospheric CO_2 (in ppm) and percent decrease of CO_2 at 12 sites in the city of Kolkata during 2019 and 2020

| SITES | COORDINATES | ATMOSPHERIC CO_2 (PPM) | | % DECREASE OF CO_2 |
		2 APRIL, 2019	24 APRIL, 2020	
Howrah station Crossing	22°34′49.4″N; 88°20′33.9″E	413	255	38.26
Moulali	22°33′40.2″N; 88°22′04.7″E	407	232	43.00
Sealdah	22°34′08.3″N; 88°22′13.4″E	410	224	45.37

(*Continued*)

TABLE 7.1 (*Continued*)   Level of atmospheric CO_2 (in ppm) and percent decrease of CO_2 at 12 sites in the city of Kolkata during 2019 and 2020

| SITES | COORDINATES | ATMOSPHERIC CO_2 (PPM) | | % DECREASE OF CO_2 |
		2 APRIL, 2019	24 APRIL, 2020	
Maniktala Crossing	22°35′05.8″N; 88°22′29.4″E	398	233	41.46
Deshbandhu Park	22°35′48.9″N; 88°22′38.6″E	338	255	24.56
Tala Park	22°36′26.8″N; 88°22′55.0″E	386	259	32.90

7.2.1 Reason for Such Observations

The nationwide lockdown has brought significant changes in almost all environmental parameters. The complete shutdown of daily operations, industrial units, transportation, businesses, markets, official establishments, educational institutions, entertainment units, amusement parks and hotels, restaurants, and other commercial ventures have significantly reduced the consumption of fossil fuels and subsequently emission of carbon dioxide. This has resulted in the major changes in CO_2 profile of the region.

The streets of the thickly populated and urbanized city of Kolkata are deserted after authorities implemented a strict lockdown. The normally bustling pubs, bars, markets, shopping malls, and theaters have been closed, and people have been told to stay in their homes. Those who are able to do so are hold up at home, practicing social distancing and working remotely.

It is all aimed at controlling the spread of COVID-19 and hopefully reducing the death toll. Similar picture was seen in New York. Compared with 2019, the levels of pollution in New York have reduced by nearly 50% because of the measures to restrict the spread of the virus (https://www.bbc.com/future/article/20200326-covid-19-the-impact-of-coronavirus-on-the-environment).

In the present study, it is seen that the decreased percentage of CO_2 in Kolkata ranged from 24.56 (at Deshbandhu Park) to 45.37 (at Sealdah station) (Figures 7.1 and 7.2). Analysis of Variance (ANOVA) showed a significant decrease between years but not between stations (Table 7.2). The variation in the CO_2 level between years can be substantiated by COVID-19 pandemic,

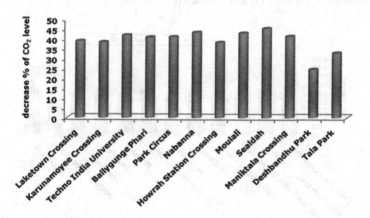

FIGURE 7.2 Spatiotemporal variation of atmospheric CO_2 (in ppm) in the study areas.

TABLE 7.2 ANOVA showing the variations of atmospheric CO_2 between sites and years in the city of Kolkata

SOURCE OF VARIATION	SS	DF	MS	F	P-VALUE	F_{CRIT}
Between sites	1797.458	11	163.4053	0.442347	0.904056	2.81793
Between years	145,860	1	145,860	394.851	5.73E-10	4.844336
Error	4063.458	11	369.4053			

but the apparent variation between sites as highlighted in Figure 7.1 (not statistically significant as revealed from Table 7.2) is attributed to existing vegetation in the site along with anthropogenic activities of various dimensions (Figure 7.3).

Sites such as Deshbandhu Park and Tala Park already have a good patch of vegetation with species such as *Mangifera indica, Delonix regia, Peltophorum pterocarpum, Ficus benghalensis, Azadirachta indica,* and *Ficus religiosa,* and hence the average CO_2 in the atmosphere was not very high during April 2019, due to which the final CO_2 value recorded during April 2020 did not show much difference unlike other sites of the city. The role of urban vegetation in storing carbon was already cited by several researchers in and around the present study area (Mitra et al., 2012; Mitra and Zaman, 2014; Banerjee et al., 2015; Mitra and Zaman, 2015; Mitra et al., 2015; Mitra et al., 2016; Agarwal 2017; Mitra, 2019; Pal et al., 2019). The overall results strongly speak in favor of the regulatory influence of COVID-19 connected lockdown in slashing down the CO_2 level in the urban atmosphere.

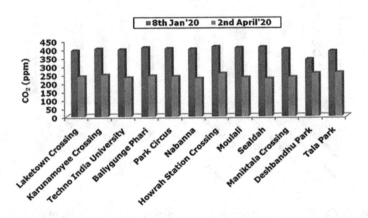

FIGURE 7.3 Percentage rates of the decreased atmospheric CO_2 level in the study areas.

REFERENCES

Agarwal, S., Pal, N., Zaman, S., and Mitra, A. (2017). "Role of mangroves in carbon sequestration: a case study from Prentice island of Indian Sundarbans." *International Journal of Basic and Applied Research*, 7 (7): 35–42.

Amirian, E.S. and Levy, J.K. (2020). "Current knowledge about the antivirals Remdesivir (GS-5734) and GS-441524 as therapeutic options for coronaviruses." *One Health*, 9: 100128.

Banerjee, R., Pramanick, P., Zaman, S., Pal, N., Mitra, S., and Mitra, A. (2015). "Impact of Urban vegetation on offsetting Carbon emission: a case study from the city of Kolkata." *Journal of Environmental Science, Computer Science and Engineering & Technology*, 4 (3): 814–818.

Barreto, M.L., Teixeira, M.G., and Carmo, E.H. (2006). "Infectious diseases epidemiology." *Journal of Epidemiol Community Health*, 60: 192–195.

Boivin, G., Abed, Y., and Pelletier, G. (2002). "Virological features and clinical manifestations associated with human metapneumovirus: a new paramyxovirus responsible for acute respiratory-tract infections in all age groups." *The Journal of Infectious Diseases*, 186: 1330–1334.

Chakravorty, A., Choudhury, M., Dutta, J., Devi, R., Deepak, K., and Rayan, R.A. (2020). "A Review on Impact of Global Climate Change on Microorganisms." *Full paper included in Chapter 6- Climate Change as a threat to Biodiversity* submitted during CLIMATE2020- THE WORLDWIDE ONLINE CLIMATE CONFERENCE. Published on weblink: https://dl4sd.org.

Chen, N., Zhou, M., Dong, X., et al. (2020). "Epidemiological and clinical characteristics of 99 cases of 2019 novel coronavirus pneumonia in Wuhan China: a descriptive study." *Lancet* (London, England), 395: 507–513.

Costa, M., and Klein, C.B. (2006). "Toxicity and carcinogenicity of chromium compounds in humans." *Critical Reviews in Toxicology*, 36(2): 155–163.

Dominguez, S.R., O'Shea, T.J., Oko, L.M., and Holmes, K.V. (2007). "Detection of group 1 coronaviruses in bats in North America." *Emerging Infectious Diseases*, 13(9): 1295–1300.

Dutta, J., Amin, G., Zaman, S., and Mitra, A. (2017). "Seasonal pattern of heavy metals levels in vegetable and fish species collected from East Kolkata Wetlands (EKW)." *International Journal for Innovative Research in Multidisciplinary Field*. ISSN: 2455-0620.

Dutta, J., Roy Chowdhury, G., and Mitra, A. (2017). "Bioaccumulation of toxic heavy metals in the edible fishes of Eastern Kolkata Wetlands (EKW): the designated Ramsar site of West Bengal, India." *International Journal of Aquaculture and Fishery Sciences*, 3(1): 18–20. ISSN 2455-8400.

Dutta, J., Zaman, S., and Mitra, A. (2018). "Are We Poisoned Every Day: How Much is Too Much?" *Paper Presented during the 2nd National Conference on Progresses in Bioengineering and Environmental Management (NCPBEM) 2018* organized by Techno India University, Salt lake, West Bengal during May 11–12, 2018.

Dutta, J., Zaman, S., and Mitra, A. (2019). "Are we taking poison every day?" *Indian Journal of Environmental Protection*, 39(3): 283–289. ISSN: 0253 7141.

Dutta, J., Sen, T., Thakur, T. K. and Mitra, A. (2020). Lead and Cadmium induced toxicity on environment and human health with special reference to peri-urban Ramsar site of India. In (Ed.) *Environment and Natural Resource Management: Economic Outlook and Opinion.* Apple Academic Press (Accepted).

Englund, J., Feuchtinger, T., and Ljungman, P. (2011). "Viral infections in immuno-compromised patients. Section 1: viral infections. ASBMT." *Biology of Blood Marrow Transplant,* 17: S2–S5.

Flora, G., Gupta, D., and Tiwari, A. (2012). "Toxicity of lead: a review with recent updates." *InterdiscipToxicology,* 5(2): 47–58.

Gautret, P., Lagier, J.C., Parola, P., et al. (2020a). "Hydroxychloroquine and azithro-mycin as a treatment of COVID-19: results of an open-label non-randomized clinical trial." *International Journal of Antimicrobial Agents,* 56(1): 105949.

Gautret, P., Lagier, J.C., Parola, P., et al. (2020b). Hydroxychloroquine-Azithromycin and COVID-19. Available at https://www.mediterranee-infection.com/wp-content/uploads/2020/03/COVID-IHU-2-1.pdf. 2020 Mar 30.

Guan, W.-j., Ni, Z.-y., Hu, Y., et al., (2020). "Clinical characteristics of 2019 novel coronavirus infection in China." 2020.02.06.20020974.

Hansen, J.C., and Dasher, G. (1997). "Organic mercury: an environmental threat to the health of dietary exposed societies?" *Reviews on Environmental Health,* 12 (2): 107–116.

Hoffmann, M., Kleine-Weber, H., Krüger, N., Müller, M., Drosten, C., and Pöhlmann, S. (2020). "The novel coronavirus 2019 (2019-nCoV) uses the SARS-coronavirus receptor ACE2 and the cellular protease TMPRSS2 for entry into target cells." *bioRxiv* preprint DOI: 10.1101/2020.01.31.929042.

Huang, C., Wang, Y., Li, Y., et al. (2020). "Clinical features of patients infected with 2019 novel coronavirus in Wuhan China." *Lancet (London, England),* 395: 497–506.

Jin, X., Lian, J. S., Hu, J. H., Gao, J., Zheng, L., Zhang, Y. M., Hao, S. R., Jia, H. Y., Cai, H., Zhang, X. L., Yu, G. D., Xu, K. J., Wang, X. Y., Gu, J. Q., Zhang, S. Y., Ye, C. Y., Jin, C. L., Lu, Y. F., Yu, X., Yu, X. P., ... Yang, Y. (2020). Epidemiological, clinical and virological characteristics of 74 cases of coronavirus-infected disease 2019 (COVID-19) with gastrointestinal symp-toms. *Gut,* 69(6), 1002–1009. DOI: 10.1136/gutjnl-2020-320926.

Kumar-M, P., Mishra, S., Jha, D.K. et al. (2020). Coronavirus disease (COVID-19) and the liver: a comprehensive systematic review and meta-analysis. *Hepatology International.* DOI: 10.1007/s12072-020-10071-9.

Le, D.H., Bloom, S.A., Nguyen, Q.H., Maloney, S.A., Le, Q.M., Leitmeyer, K.C., Bach, H.A., Reynolds, M.G., Montgomery, J.M., Comer, J.A., Horby, P.W., and Plant, A.J. (2004). "Lack of SARS transmission among public hospital workers Vietnam." *Emerging Infectious Diseases,* 10 (2): 265–268.

Lipsitch, M., Cohen, T., Cooper, B., et al. (2003). "Transmission dynamics and control of severe acute respiratory syndrome." *Science (New York, NY),* 300: 1966–1970.

Liu, Y., Gayle, A.A., Wilder-Smith, A., and Rocklov, J. (2020). "The reproductive number of COVID-19 is higher compared to SARS coronavirus." *Journal of Travel Medicine,* 27(2).

Mahaffey K.R. (1990). "Environmental lead toxicity: nutrition as a component of intervention." *Environ Health Perspect,* 89: 75–78.

Majumder, M.S., Rivers, C., Lofgren, E., and Fisman, D. (2014). "Estimation of MERS-coronavirus reproductive number and case fatality rate for the Spring 2014 Saudi Arabia outbreak: insights from publicly available data." *PLoS Currents*, 6.

Mallik, A., Dutta, J., Sultana, P., and Mitra, A. (2017). "Bioaccumulation pattern of heavy metals in vegetables collected from selected areas in and around Kolkata city (India)." *International Journal of Higher Education and Research (IJHER)*, 7 (2): 121–134. ISSN: 2277 260X.

Milano, F., Campbell, A.P., Guthrie, K.A., and Kuypers, J. (2010). "Human rhinovirus and coronavirus detection among allogeneic hematopoietic stem cell transplantation recipients." *Blood*, 115: 2088–2094.

Mitra, A. (2019). *Estuarine Pollution in the Lower Gangetic Delta*. Published by Springer International Publishing, ISBN 978-3-319-93305-4, XVI: 371.

Mitra, A., Bagchi, J., Thakur, S., Parkhi, U.S., Debnath, S., Pramanick, P., and Zaman, S. (2015). "Carbon sequestration in Bhubaneswar city of Odisha, India." *International Journal of Innovative Research in Science, Engineering and Technology*, 4 (8): 6942–6947.

Mitra, A., Rudra, T., Guha, A., Ray, A., Pramanick, P., Pal, N., and Zaman, S. (2016). "Ecosystem service of *Avicennia alba* in terms of carbon sequestration." *Journal of Environmental Science, Computer Science and Engineering & Technology*, 5 (1), 155–160

Mitra, A., Sengupta, K., and Banerjee, K. (2012). "Spatial and temporal trends in biomass and carbon sequestration potential of *Sonneratia apetala* Buch-Ham in Indian Sundarbans." *Proceedings of the National Academy of Sciences, India, Section B: Biological Sciences*, 82 (2): 317–323 (SPRINGER DOI 10.1007/s40011-012-0021-5).

Mitra, A., and Zaman, S. (2014). *Carbon Sequestration by Coastal Floral Community, India*. Published by The Energy and Resources Institute (TERI) TERI Press. ISBN 978-81-7993-551-4.

Mitra, A., and Zaman, S. (2015). *Blue Carbon Reservoir of the Blue Planet*. Published by Springer, ISBN 978-81-322-2106-7 (Springer DOI 10.1007/978-81-322-2107-4).

Mitra, A. and Zaman, S. (2016). *Basics of Marine and Estuarine Ecology*. Published by Springer, ISBN 978-81-322-2705-2.

Molina, J.M., Delaugerre, C., Goff, J.L., et al. (2020). "No evidence of rapid antiviral clearance or clinical benefit with the combination of hydroxychloroquine and azithromycin in patients with severe COVID-19 infection." *Médecine et Maladies Infectieuses*, 50 (4): 384.

Pal, N., Mitra, A., Zaman, S. and Mitra, A. (2019). "Natural oxygen counters in Indian Sundarbans, the mangrove dominated World Heritage Site." *Parana Journal of Science and Education*, 5 (2): 6–13.

Panda, K.K., Lenka, M., and Panda, B.B., (1992). "Monitoring and assessment of mercury pollution in the vicinity of a chloralkali plant. II. Plantavailability, tissue-concentration and genotoxicity of mercury from agricultural soil contaminated with solid waste assessed in barley(Hordeumvulgare L.)." *Environmental Pollution*, 76 (1): 33–42.

Peret, T.C., Boivin, G., and Li, Y. (2002). Characterization of human metapneumoviruses isolated from patients in North America. *The Journal of Infectious Diseases*,185: 1660–1663. [PMC free article] [PubMed] [Google Scholar]

Remais, J. (2010). "Modelling environmentally-mediated infectious diseases of humans: transmission dynamics of schistosomiasis in China." *Advances in Experimental Medicine and Biology*, 673: 79–98.

Schenk, T., Strahm, B., Kontny, U., Hufnagel, M., Neumann-Haefelin, D., and Falcone, V. (2007). "Disseminated bocavirus infection after stem cell transplant." *Emerging Infectious Diseases,* 13: 1425–1427.

Sharma, S., and Bhattacharya, A. (2017). "Drinking water contamination and treatment techniques." *Applied Water Science* 7: 1043–1067.

Tchounwou, P. B., Yedjou, C. G., Patlolla, A. K., and Sutton, D. J. (2012). Heavy metal toxicity and the environment. *Experientia supplementum*, 101: 133–164.

Wang, Z., Chai, L., Wang, Y., Yang, Z., Wang, H., and Wu, X. (2011). "Potential health risk of arsenic and cadmium in groundwater near Xiang jiang river, China: a case study for risk assessment and management of toxic substances." *Environmental Monitoring and Assessment*, 175: 167–173.

Wani, A.L., Ara, A. and Usmani, J.A. (2015). "Lead toxicity: a review." *InterdiscipToxicol*, 8(2): 55–64.

WHO. (2020). Coronavirus Disease 2019(COVID-19) Situation Report–46.

Woolhouse, M.E. (2002). "Population biology of emerging and re-emerging pathogens." *Trends Microbiology*, 10: S3–S7 DOI: 10.1016/S0966-842X(02)02428-9.

Woolhouse, M.E., and Gowtage-Sequeria, S. (2005). "Host range and emerging and reemerging pathogens." *Emerging Infectious Diseases* 11: 1842–1847.

Wrapp, D., Wang, N., Corbett, K.S., et al. (2020). "Cryo-EM structure of the 2019-nCoV spike in the prefusion conformation." Science 367(6483): 1260–1263.

Wu, J.T., Leung, K., Leung, G.M. (2020). "Nowcasting and forecasting the potential domestic and international spread of the 2019-nCoV outbreak originating in Wuhan China: a modelling study." The Lancet, 395(10225): P689–697.

Wu, Z., and McGoogan, J.M. (2020). "Characteristics of and important lessons from the coronavirus disease 2019 (COVID-19) outbreak in China: summary of a report of 72314 cases from the Chinese center for disease control and prevention." *The Journal of the American Medical Association. JAMA*. 323(13): 1239–1242. DOI: 10.1001/jama.2020.2648

Wu, A., Peng, Y., Huang, B., Ding, X., Wang, X., Niu, P., Meng, J., Zhu, Z., Zhang, Z., Wang, J., Sheng, J., Quan, L., Xia, Z., Tan, W., Cheng, G., and Jiang, T. (2020). "Genome composition and divergence of the novel coronavirus (2019-nCoV) originating in China." *Cell Host Microbe*. 27(3): 325–328. DOI: 10.1016/j.chom.2020.02.001. Epub 2020 Feb 7.

Wu, J., Song, S., Cao, H. C., and Li, L. J. (2020). Liver diseases in COVID-19: Etiology, treatment and prognosis. *World journal of gastroenterology*, 26(19): 2286–2293.

Xu, X., Chen, P., Wang, J., Feng, J., Zhou, H., Li, X. (2020). Evolution of the novel coronavirus from the ongoing Wuhan outbreak and modeling of its spike protein for risk of human transmission. *Science China Life Sciences*, 63(3):457–460.

Zahir, F., Rizwi, S.J., Haq, S.K., and Khan, R.H. (2005). "Low dose mercury toxicity and human health." *Environmental Toxicology and Pharmacology*.

Zhang, M.Q., Zhu, Y.C., and Deng, R.W. (2002). "Evaluation of mercury emissions to the atmosphere from coal combustion, China." *Ambio*, 31 (6): 482–484.

WEBLINK

https://edition.cnn.com/ 2020/04/02/health/aerosol-coronavirus-spread whitehouseletter/
index.html

https://www.bbc.com/future/article/ 20200326-covid-19-the-impact-of-coronavirus-
on-the-environment

Trends in Water Pollution during the COVID-19 Lockdown Phase

8

8.1 STATUS OF BRACKISH WATER PHYTOPLANKTON DURING COVID-19 LOCKDOWN PHASE

Phytoplankton community represents free-floating, microscopic floral entities that thrive luxuriantly within the photic zone of the ocean, estuaries, and different aquatic systems. It encompasses both prokaryotic and eukaryotic species. The phytoplankton community is a key player in maintaining the nutrient and energy flow through marine and estuarine food webs. One of the major challenges for aquatic ecologists is to understand the natural processes and anthropogenic factors that regulate the standing biomass of phytoplankton in pelagic ecosystems. Understanding these processes would improve our ability to regulate/control nuisance and toxic algal blooms, maintain the esthetics of surface water bodies, protect drinking water supplies, and improve fisheries production (Vollenweider, 1976; Carpenter et al., 1985; McQueen et al., 1986; Carmichael, 1994; Pauly and Christensen, 1995; Brett and Goldman, 1996, 1997; Falconer, 1999; Micheli, 1999). Phytoplankton is the foundation of the aquatic food cycle, meaning that they are the primary producers (Vargas et al., 2006).

The fish resources of the nation, which are directly linked to the economic profile of the country, is dependent on the phytoplankton stock as they are primary producers of the aquatic system and transfer energy to members of higher trophic levels such as fishes and other commercially important aquatic species by serving as their major food sources. The current analysis is, therefore, an attempt to assess their status during the COVID-19 lockdown phase, when all the pollution sources have been cut-off, leading to improved environmental quality (Mitra et al., 2020).

The analytical results show that the standing stock of phytoplankton in the select station is the highest in April 2020 compared to that of April 2019 as highlighted in Figure 8.1.

The phytoplankton at the base of the aquatic food pyramid is exposed to threats of various categories arising from industrial and domestic discharges. The suspended particulate matter (SPM) and oil film associated with aquatic ecosystem prevents the solar energy from penetrating the water column, thereby posing a negative impact on phytoplankton. This type of stress is common in the estuarine water of Indian Sundarbans due to continuous movement of passenger vessels, fishing trawlers, ships, and oil tankers along the navigation route. In addition to this, the industries situated along the Hooghly estuary also add a substantial volume of suspended particles in the water body, thus retarding the growth of the tiny producer community (Mitra, 2013; Mitra and Zaman, 2014; Mitra and Zaman, 2015; Mitra and Zaman, 2016; Mitra, 2019). The COVID-19 phase, however, turned the picture of the environment (Mitra et al., 2020). Due to the lockdown imposed by the Central and state governments, the discharges from industries and tourism units have been cut off. In addition, the water transport system has also ceased due to which the stress on this tiny producer community has been eliminated. This is reflected by the higher standing stock of phytoplankton during April 2020 (430.63×10^5/L), compared to that of April 2019 (226.75×10^5/L) and April 2018 (219.03×10^5/L) as shown in Figure 8.1 This increase in standing stock has a high probability for the acceleration of estuarine fish resources in the years to come.

The results indicate that the COVID-19 lockdown phase has accelerated the growth of phytoplankton species in the brackish water system along the Hooghly estuary, probably due to the complete removal of the stress from pollution from point and nonpoint sources. Thus, the COVID-19 lockdown process has positively impacted the biodiversity of the aquatic ecosystem.

Figure 8.1 illustrates how various anthropogenic stressors negatively impact the phytoplankton communities. The constant movement of passenger and industrial vessels as well as the factories along the Hooghly Industrial Belt results in the pollution of the brackish water system along the Hooghly estuary. The resultant SPM and oil films contaminating the aquatic ecosystem prevents proper penetration of solar radiation, thereby negatively affecting the phytoplankton communities. Due to the government-mandated

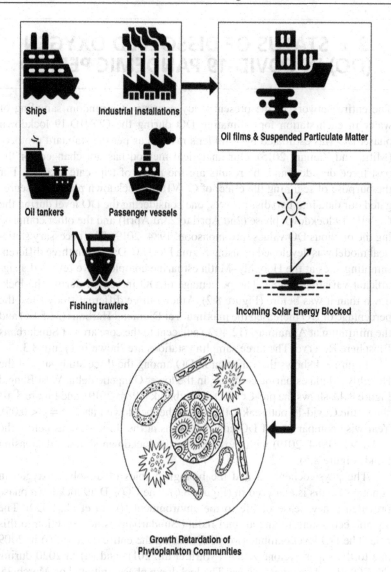

Ships

Industrial installations

Oil films & Suspended Particulate Matter

Oil tankers

Passenger vessels

Fishing trawlers

Incoming Solar Energy Blocked

Growth Retardation of Phytoplankton Communities

FIGURE 8.1 Impact of COVID-19 lockdown on aquatic ecosystems.

lockdown, these anthropogenic stressors were significantly reduced. This reflected in the higher standing stock of phytoplankton during April 2020 as uncovered by our current analysis. This increase in the standing stock can potentially accelerate the estuarine fish resources in the coming years.

8.2 STATUS OF DISSOLVED OXYGEN (DO) IN COVID-19 PANDEMIC PERIOD

The entire network of the present study consists of a random sampling of water in each station for estimating DO during the COVID-19 lockdown phase. DO was estimated by Winkler's method as per the standard protocol (Mitra and Zaman, 2015). Our analytical method has not changed for the past three decades, and the results are the mean of triplicate analysis. For the purpose of scanning the effect of COVID-19 lockdown phase, we segregated our data into two distinct sets, one considering the DO level during the COVID-19 lockdown phase (2nd April to 23rd April) and the other comprising the previous DO values (pre-monsoon, 1984–2019). The necessary statistical model was developed by using Sigma Plot11.0. Data from three different sampling sites at the Hooghly–Matla estuarine complex have revealed a significant variation in DO. The percentage of DO increased during the lockdown than it was before (Figure 8.2). Among three different study sites, the percentage of DO increased the maximum at Diamond Harbour (38.54%) and the minimum at Ajmalmari (12.40%) adjacent to the core area of Sundarbans Biosphere Reserve. The three sampling stations are shown in Figure 8.3.

Figure 8.4 shows the variation in DO among the three study sites at the Hooghly–Matla estuarine complex, in the lower Gangetic delta, West Bengal Figure 8.4A shows the pre-COVID-19 outbreak (1984–2019), and Figure 8.4B shows the Covid-19 outbreak followed by the lockdown phase ($* = p < 0.05$). Year-wise comparison of DO concentrations at the three stations before the lockdown (1984–2019) with those during the lockdown shows a decreasing trend (Figure 8.5).

The physicochemical and the biological roles of dissolved oxygen in aquatic systems is analyzed in (Figure 8.6). The COVID-19 lockdown phase provided a new lease of life to the environment (Mitra et al., 2020). The aquatic ecosystem in and around Indian Sundarbans is no exception to this rule. The DO level exhibits two peaks during the entire data set: (i) in 2009 due to the super cyclone AILA (Mitra et al., 2011) and (ii) in 2020 during the COVID-19 lockdown phase. The lockdown phase, initiated on March 25, 2020, completely ceased all the industrial operations and water transport, which ultimately improved the estuarine water quality as revealed by the hike in DO values. This increase has several positive implications particularly in the domain of sustaining the fish resources of the estuarine system.

(a)
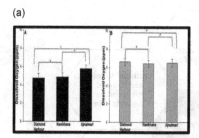

(b)
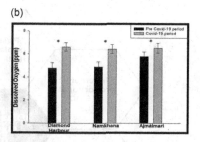

FIGURE 8.2 (a) and (b) shows the prominent differences in DO concentration before and after the lockdown.

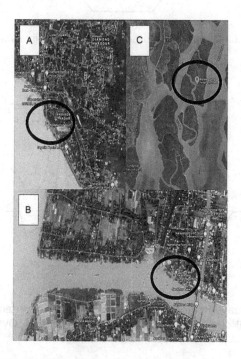

FIGURE 8.3 GPS location of three sampling sites in the Hooghly–Matla estuarine complex A. Diamond Harbour, B. Namkhana, and C. Ajmalmari.

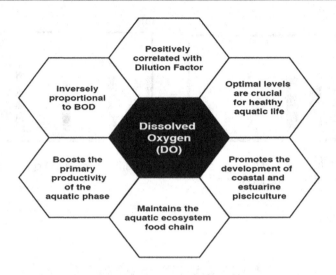

FIGURE 8.4   Multifarious role of dissolved oxygen (DO) in aquatic ecosystems.

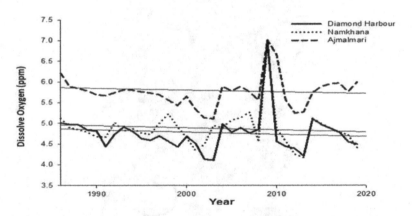

FIGURE 8.5   Year-wise trends in dissolved oxygen (DO) concentration at three stations in the Hooghly–Matla estuarine complex before COVID (1984–2019) and during the COVID-19 lockdown phase (April, 2020).

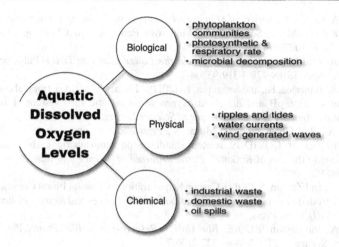

FIGURE 8.6 Physicochemical and biological roles of dissolved oxygen (DO) in aquatic ecosystems.

REFERENCES

Brett, M.T., and Goldman, C.R. (1996). "A meta-analysis of the freshwater trophic cascade." *Proceedings of the National Academy of Sciences of the United States of America*, 93: 7723–7726.

Brett, M.T. and Goldman, C.R. (1997). "Consumer versus resource control in freshwater pelagic food webs." *Science*, 275: 384–386.

Carmichael, W.W. (1994). "The toxins of cyanobacteria. "*Scientific American*: 78–102.

Carpenter, S.R., Kitchell, J.F., and Hodgson, J.R. (1985). "Cascading trophic interactions and lake productivity." *BioScience*, 35: 634–639.

Falconer, I.R. (1999). "An overview of problems caused by toxic blue–green algae (cyanobacteria) in drinking and recreational water." *Environmental Toxicology*, 14: 5–12.

McQueen, D.J., Post, J.R., and Mills, E.L. (1986). "Trophic relationships in freshwater pelagic ecosystems." *Canadian Journal of Fisheries & Aquatic Sciences*, 43: 1571–1581.

Micheli, F. (1999). "Eutrophication, fisheries, and consumer resource dynamics in marine pelagic ecosystems." *Science*, 285: 1396–1398.

Mitra, A. (2013). *Sensitivity of Mangrove Ecosystem to Changing Climate.* Springer. DOI: A. Mitra, Sensitivity of Mangrove Ecosystem to Changing Climate, DOI 10.1007/978-81-322-1509-7_1.

Mitra, A. (2019). *Estuarine Pollution in the Lower Gangetic Delta.* Published by Springer. ISBN 978-3-319-93304-7.

Mitra, A., Banerjee, K., and Sengupta, K. (2011). "Impact of AILA, a tropical cyclone on salinity, pH and dissolved oxygen of an aquatic sub- system of Indian Sundarbans." *National Academy of Science Letters,* 81 (II): 198–205.

Mitra, A., Ray Chaudhury, T., Mitra, A., Pramanick, P., and Zaman, S. (2020). "Impact of COVID-19 related shutdown on atmospheric carbon dioxide level in the city of Kolkata." *Parana Journal of Science and Education,* 6(3): 84–92.

Mitra, A., and Zaman, S. (2014). Carbon Sequestration by Coastal Floral Community: A ground Zero observation on blue carbon. *The Energy and Resources Institute (TERI)* TERI Press.

Mitra, A., and Zaman, S. (2015). *Blue Carbon Reservoir of the Blue Planet.* Published by Springer. ISBN 978-81-322-2106-7.

Mitra, A. and Zaman, S. (2016). *Basics of Marine and Estuarine Ecology.* Published by Springer. ISBN 978-81-322-2705-2.

Pauly, D. and Christensen, V. (1995). "Primary production required to sustain global fisheries." *Nature,* 374: 255–257.

Vargas. C.A., Escribano, R. and Poulet, S. (2006). "Phytoplankton food quality determines time windows for successful zooplankton reproductive pulses." *Ecology,* 8: 2992–2999.

Vollenweider, R.A. (1976). "Advances in defining critical loading levels for phosphorus in lake eutrophication." *Memorie dell' Istituto Italiano di Idrobiologia,* 33: 53–83.

Frequently Asked Questions about COVID-19

9

COVID-19 is a completely new disease, and very little is known about the behavior of SARS-CoV-2 and the course this disease. Scientists around the world are working tirelessly with the sole aim of developing a safe and effective cure for COVID-19. Until then, undertaking appropriate safety and hygiene measures is the key to stay safe. In any pandemic situation, misinformation and rumor spreads more quickly than the pathogen itself, which can be just as dangerous. We all have a role to play in protecting ourselves and others. Knowing the facts about COVID-19 helps stop the spread of rumors and the disease. Here are 10 most frequently asked questions about COVID-19 as per the report of the World Health Organization.

1. **Can I Wear Mask during Exercise?:** The World Health Organization does not recommend wearing mask during exercise. During exercise, the body's need for oxygen increases, and wearing mask interferes with the breathing process. In addition, during exercise, sweat makes the mask wet, which promotes the growth of microorganisms (WHO, 2020).
2. **Can Wearing Medical Masks Cause CO_2 Intoxication, and O_2 Deficiency?:** Properly wearing medical masks (surgical masks) does not cause CO_2 intoxication or O_2 deficiency. Reuse of disposable medical masks is not recommended (WHO, 2020).
3. **Can COVID-19 Be Transmitted through Shoes?:** The chances of COVID-19 being transmitted through shoes is very low. Since dirt,

mud, and other waste materials from the road may get stuck to the bottom of the shoes and might carry germs to the home, it is a good practice to keep shoes outside before entering a room. Maintaining proper hygiene is the key to safety (WHO, 2020).

4. **Does Alcohol Consumption Provide Protection against COVID-19?:** Consumption of alcohol does not provide protection against COVID-19. Alcohol is an addictive substance and causes chronic diseases such as hypertension, cardiovascular disease, miscarriage and stillbirth, cancer and degeneration of mental health. Alcohol weakens the body's immune system (ability to fight infections) and makes an individual more vulnerable to infectious diseases (CDC, 2019; WHO, 2020).

5. **Does Tobacco Consumption Provide Protection against COVID-19?:** Consumption of tobacco does not provide protection against COVID-19. Tobacco is an addictive substance and causes chronic diseases such as cancer, cardiovascular disease, diseases of the respiratory system and also weakens the body's immune system. Like alcohol, consumption of tobacco (smoking or chewing, etc.) makes an individual vulnerable to infectious or other degenerative diseases or even death (CDC, 2020; WHO, 2020).

6. **Can COVID-19 Be Detected Using Thermal Scanners?:** Thermal scanners are designed to detect changes in temperature. For example, fever causes a rise in body temperature, which can be recorded using a thermal scanner. But a thermal scanner cannot detect whether a person is infected with COVID-19 or not (WHO, 2020).

7. **Does Flies or Mosquitoes Spread COVID-19?:** There are no studies or evidence that suggests SARS-CoV-2 can be transmitted through mosquito bites or flies (WHO, 2020). But since flies and mosquitoes are associated with other kinds of infectious diseases such as malaria and dengue, maintaining proper hygiene and implementing protective measures against these organisms is a healthy practice.

8. **Does Antibiotics Cure COVID-19?:** COVID-19 is a disease caused by a coronavirus known as SARS-CoV-2. Antibiotics do not kill or stop the growth of viruses. Antibiotics are only effective against bacterial diseases. So taking antibiotics does not cure COVID-19.

9. **Does Flu or Pneumonia Vaccines Provide Protection against COVID-19?:** Vaccines for pneumonia does not provide protection against COVID-19. Scientists around the world are working

tirelessly with the sole aim of developing safe and effective vaccines for COVID-19 (WHO, 2020).

10. **Is Consuming and Spraying Bleach or Disinfectant on the Body Dangerous?:** Methanol, ethanol, or disinfectants are highly poisonous substances and its consumption leads to disability or even death. Disinfectants are used to disinfect fomites. Spraying of disinfectant on the body is not recommended as the chemicals damage the skin and causes skin disease. Personal protective equipment such as eye protection, gloves, mask, or apron should be used while handling these kinds of poisonous disinfectants. These poisonous chemicals should be kept away from the reach of children and pets (WHO, 2020).

When in doubt about the authenticity of any information related to COVID-19, the authors recommend that the readers follow the official websites of the World Health Organization (www.who.int), Centers for Disease Control and Prevention (www.cdc.gov) and other official government websites regulated by the ministry of health in their respective countries. These organizations provide authentic, evidence-based and up-to-date information periodically.

REFERENCES

Alcohol and Public Health. (2019, December 30). Centers for Disease Control and Prevention. Available at https://www.cdc.gov/alcohol/fact-sheets/alcohol-use.htm. Accessed on July 12, 2020.

Coronavirus disease (COVID-19). (2020, June 4). Advice for the Public: Mythbusters. World Health Organization. Available at https://www.who.int/emergencies/diseases/novel-coronavirus-2019/advice-for-public. Accessed on July 12, 2020.

Smoking and Tobacco Use. (2020, April 28). Centers for Disease Control and Prevention. Available at https://www.cdc.gov/tobacco/basic_information/health_effects/index.htm. Accessed on July 12, 2020.